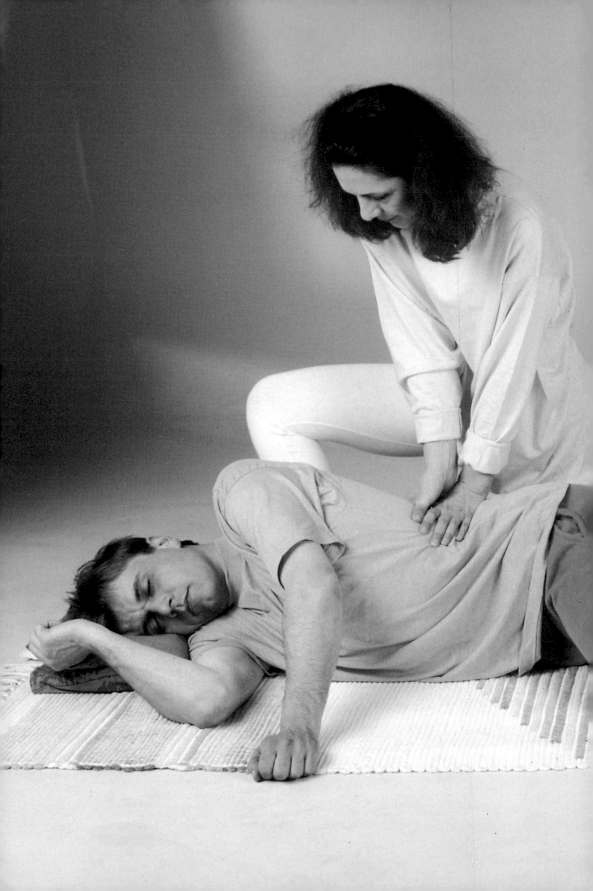

THE BOOK OF
SHIATSU

Paul Lundberg

Photography by Fausto Dorelli

A GAIA ORIGINAL

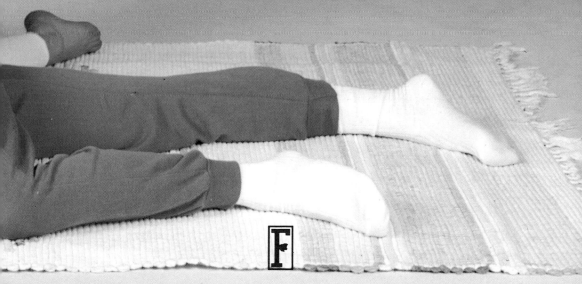

A Fireside Book
Published by Simon & Schuster Inc.
New York   London   Toronto   Sydney   Tokyo   Singapore

A GAIA ORIGINAL

Conceived by	Joss Pearson
Editorial	Eleanor Lines Katherine Pate
Design	Dave Thorp
Illustration	Sheilagh Noble Paula Cox
Direction	Joss Pearson Patrick Nugent

FIRESIDE
Simon & Schuster Building
Rockefeller Center
1230 Avenue of the Americas
New York, New York 10020

Typeset by Tradespools Ltd, Somerset, UK
Reproduction by David Bruce Graphics Ltd, London
Printed in Singapore by Imago

10 9 8 7 6 5 4

Library of Congress Cataloging-in-publication Data
Lundberg, Paul.
  The book of shiatsu / Paul Lundberg : photography by Fausto
Dorelli.
   p. cm.
  ''A Gaia original''
  ''A Fireside book''
  ISBN 0-671-74488-7
  1. Acupressure.
RM723.A27L86 1992   91-18484
615.8'22—dc20   CIP

Caution

The techniques, ideas, and suggestions in this book are to be used at the reader's sole discretion and risk. Always observe the cautions given, and consult a doctor if you are in doubt about a medical condition.

  Shiatsu is very safe when performed according to the principles described in this book. It can be very effective in relieving chronic discomforts as well as many minor acute ailments and illnesses. Three medical conditions require cautions: pregnancy, high blood pressure, and epilepsy.

  In pregnancy, observe the cautions on page 176 and throughout the book. Do not apply strong pressure to the top of the shoulders. Avoid points LI 4 (see p. 96) and Sp 6 (see p. 103), and the Yin Channels (Spleen, Kidney, and Liver) below the knees.

  For people with high blood pressure or epilepsy, do not give shiatsu on top of the head. However, work on the limbs, especially the legs and feet, is beneficial and safe. Avoid leaning heavily on elderly or infirm people — especially those with arthritis or osteoporosis (brittle bones); treat them in the sitting position, described on pages 178–185.

HOW TO USE THIS BOOK

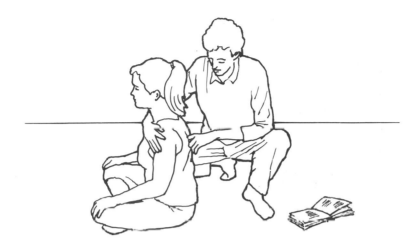

The Book of Shiatsu is a comprehensive introduction to the use of gentle manipulation and hand pressure to bring health and vitality to your life. It is for the interested novice as well as the shiatsu student; for givers and receivers of shiatsu alike. **Part One** illustrates and describes in detail the fundamentals of Oriental medicine, prepares you physically and mentally for beginning shiatsu, and explains the techniques to use and the principles to follow. It ends with a simple shiatsu routine. **Part Two** presents three more detailed routines that, together, cover all the pathways of your work on the body. The chapters in Part Two describe in detail the functions of every Organ, as well as the symptoms associated with them. **Part Three** extends your knowledge into the area of diagnosis, and encourages you to adapt your work to suit the particular needs of your shiatsu partner.

Initial capital letters on some anatomical words indicate their Oriental meaning, which has wider connotations than the same words in the West. See page 80 for a fuller explanation.

A note on clothing
A shiatsu session can take place with both participants comfortably dressed. No special clothing is necessary.

Observe the cautions given on the facing page.

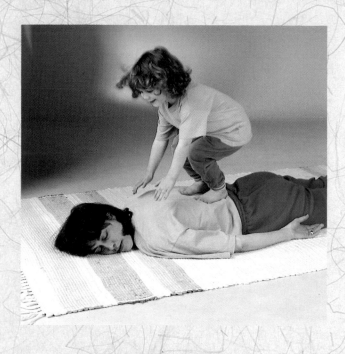

FOREWORD

Western medicine provides many remedies for the diseases and problems we encounter in our daily lives, but by concentrating almost exclusively on illness and failing to address the essence of health, modern medicine falls far short of our needs.

Eastern medicine posits a "life force" or "energy" (referred to variously as Ki, Chi, or Prana) that defines us as living beings. The characteristics and condition of this vital energy comprise the essence of our state of wellness or illness. Thus Eastern medicine concentrates on maintaining Ki in an optimal condition – or restoring it back to such a condition – as the heart of the practice of medicine. The concept that we possess internal resources on which we can draw to sustain our health has slowly been gaining acceptance.

Through manual manipulation of the body in conjunction with the use of natural substances, such as herbs, Eastern medicine aims to uncover all the resources we have within ourselves that contribute to a state of wellbeing. Experience has shown that achieving this state produces long-term, stable results, rather than short-term, immediate relief.

Our search for health is a metaphor for our desire to understand ourselves and for that understanding to influence our lives in a positive, fulfilling manner. One method of having such an influence involves the use and practice of shiatsu.

Literally translated as "finger pressure", shiatsu is a Japanese form of body work designed to heal and promote health by influencing and improving the state of Ki in the body. The principles of shiatsu conform to natural law by respecting and utilizing the relationship we have with nature. Shiatsu capitalizes on our innate response to touch, our capacity to intuit, and our ability to exercise "mind over matter" in pursuit of an ultimate condition of wellbeing. It is with this pursuit of wellbeing in mind that *The Book of Shiatsu* is written.

Those who wish to gain a basic knowledge of shiatsu for home use will find the chapters on technique thorough, yet simple enough to follow easily. For the more advanced student of shiatsu, this book can serve as a basic text that provides an understanding of shiatsu as a total system, including theory, technique, self-help exercises, and diagnosis. The chapter on "Your Own Wellbeing" is particularly helpful for strengthening techniques. This book is also an excellent reference resource for those who already have substantial knowledge of shiatsu. The chapters on diagnostic techniques are especially helpful.

Lastly, even for those simply interested in reading about shiatsu, this book presents in a clear and concise manner, everything one needs to know to become conversant with the subject. However, true understanding comes only through practical experience. In other words, the reader should not resist the temptation to actually put into practice what he or she reads.

The degree of relaxation and ease achieved through shiatsu goes beyond inner ease. So exploit this opportunity to explore a time-honoured means of improving your sense of wellbeing by using a technique that, in various forms, has been helping people for thousands of years.

Pauline Sasaki
Director of Shiatsu Program
Connecticut Center for Massage Therapy

Contents

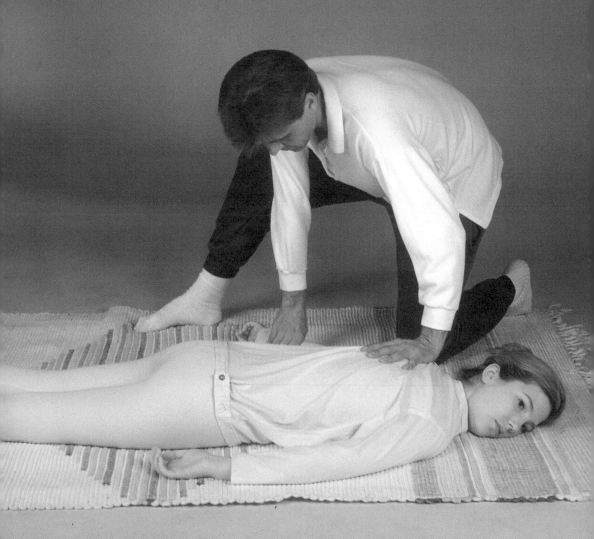

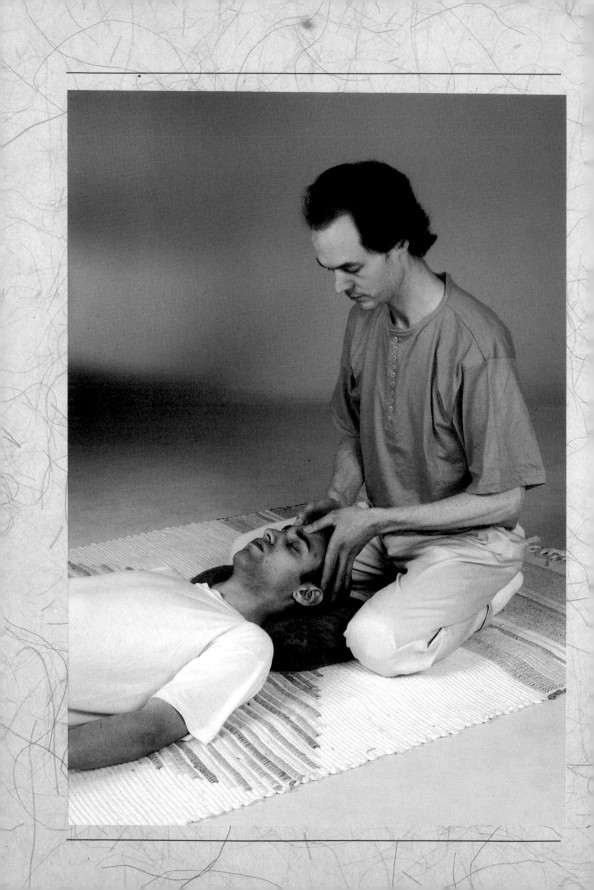

Introduction

Shiatsu is a Japanese word meaning "finger pressure". It is a new name for the oldest form of medicine – healing with hands. Everybody has the healing power of touch and responds to touch. It is a natural ability that people are now beginning to recognize again. Shiatsu uses hand pressure and manipulative techniques to adjust the body's physical structure and its natural inner energies, to help ward off illness, and maintain good health.

Shiatsu is characterized by its great simplicity. It grew from earlier forms of massage, called Anma in Japan (Anmo or Tuina in China) which use rubbing, stroking, squeezing, tapping, pushing, and pulling to influence the muscles and circulatory systems of the body. Shiatsu, by contrast, uses few techniques and to an observer it would appear that little is happening - merely a still, relaxed pressure at various points on the body with the hand or thumb, an easy leaning of the elbows or a simple rotation of a limb. It almost seems a lazy activity and, to the extent that it conserves one's energy, it is. But underneath the uncomplicated movements much is happening internally to the body's energy on a subtle level.

Subtle energy in the body

The Oriental tradition describes the world in terms of energy. All things are considered to be manifestations of a vital universal force, called "Ki" by the Japanese, "Chi", or "Qi", in China. Because of the Japanese origins of shiatsu therapy, the Japanese word Ki is used in preference to the Chinese word, Chi. Ki is the primary substance and motive force of life. It is most often described as "energy", but Ki is also synonymous with breath in the Japanese and Chinese languages. In Oriental medicine, harmony of Ki within the human body is conceived as being essential to health. All its endeavours are addressed to this end.

The aims of this book

This book is written for both "givers" and "receivers" of shiatsu. Shiatsu is for sharing with others, and you can enhance your health and your enjoyment of life by following the demonstrations illustrated in the book. By learning the basic principles of traditional Oriental medicine, you can also use your shiatsu to help when your friends or members of your family are unwell.

But the study of the treatment of disease, or individual symptoms, can lead to a limited view of shiatsu and its benefits. This book gives you a grounding in techniques and pathways for working on the body, from which you can develop your understanding of the body's "energetic" system - its network of energy. Rather than concentrating on curing diseases, you will gain a feeling for the relationship between illness and health. Shiatsu can help you to even out the swings between extremes, find an appropriate balance, and live more fully and creatively.

The development of shiatsu in Japan

Shiatsu was developed in the early part of the 20th century by a Japanese practitioner, Tamai Tempaka, who incorporated the newer Western medical knowledge of anatomy and physiology into several older methods of treatment. Originally he called it "Shiatsu Ryoho", or "finger pressure way of healing", then "Shiatsu Ho", "finger pressure method". Now known simply as "shiatsu", it was officially recognized as a therapy by the Japanese Government in 1964, so distinguishing it from the older form of traditional massage, Anma. The role of shiatsu therapists is to diagnose and treat according to the principles of Oriental medicine.

Chinese origins of shiatsu

The earliest known book of Chinese medicine is called the 'Huang Ti Nei Ching', 'The Yellow Emperor's Classic of Internal Medicine'. In it the legendary Emperor questions his physician, Ch'i Po, about problems of medicine and health among his people. In one well known passage Ch'i Po explains that different forms of medicine were developed in different regions according to the prevailing climate and the resulting constitutional problems from which people suffered. Treatment using herbs, needles and heat were attributed to Northern, Southern, Eastern, and Western regions, but development of physical therapy including massage and breathing exercise was accorded to the people of China's central region. Thus began the long association of massage and manipulative therapy with special physical exercise, breathing techniques, and healing meditations which represented the highest level of Chinese medicine. These came to be known collectively as "Tao Yin", methods for guiding the subtle energies within the body to flow smoothly. Shiatsu is the modern inheritor of this tradition. Chinese medicine was introduced to Japan by a Buddhist monk in the 6th century. The Japanese developed and refined many of its methods to suit their own physiology, temperament, and climate. In particular they developed the manual healing and diagnostic arts, evolving special techniques of abdominal diagnosis, treatment, and abdominal massage (see pp. 164-5).

Styles of shiatsu

Many early shiatsu practitioners developed their own style and some, including Tokojiro Namikoshi and Shizuto Masunaga, founded schools that helped establish shiatsu as a therapy. There are many different styles of shiatsu today. Some concentrate on "acupressure (acupuncture) points". Some emphasize more general work on the body or along the pathways of energy to influence the Ki that flows in them. Others highlight diagnostic systems, such as the "Five Element" system or the macrobiotic approach. But all of these are based in traditional Chinese medicine. This book is intended as a broadly based guide to shiatsu, drawing on the most useful and practical aspects of the different approaches, with traditional Chinese medicine as its basis. However, one particular source of inspiration should be mentioned - the "Zen" shiatsu of Shizuto Masunaga.

Zen shiatsu

Masunaga incorporated his experience of shiatsu into his studies of Western psychology and Chinese medicine; he also refined the existing methods of diagnosis. His extended system incorporated special exercises, known as "Makko Ho", to stimulate the flow of Ki, and he developed a set of guiding principles to make the techniques more effective. He called his system "Zen Shiatsu" after the simple and direct approach to spirituality of the Zen Buddhist monks in Japan.

A note on the Chinese approach to understanding the body and health

In this book, you may notice a circularity in the logic of Chinese medicine. Westerners think of cause and effect as a linear progression of ideas and events from A, through B, to C. Eastern philosophy regards events as mutually conditioned, arising together. They are not seen as distinct from the environment in which they occur. The background is as important as the foreground. An example is given here to help to clarify the difference.

A headache is not just an event in the head, according to Chinese medicine, nor is it merely a pain, or something to be stopped without regard for its origins, nor even treated on the same basis as someone else's headache. Rather, it is an obstruction of Ki, related to the overall energy patterns in the whole body of the particular individual, their circumstances, and lifestyle. Treatment might involve work on the arms or legs as well as (or instead of) the head and will bring more lasting and satisfactory changes than will an attempt to block the superficial symptoms.

Observe the cautions given facing page 5 of this book.

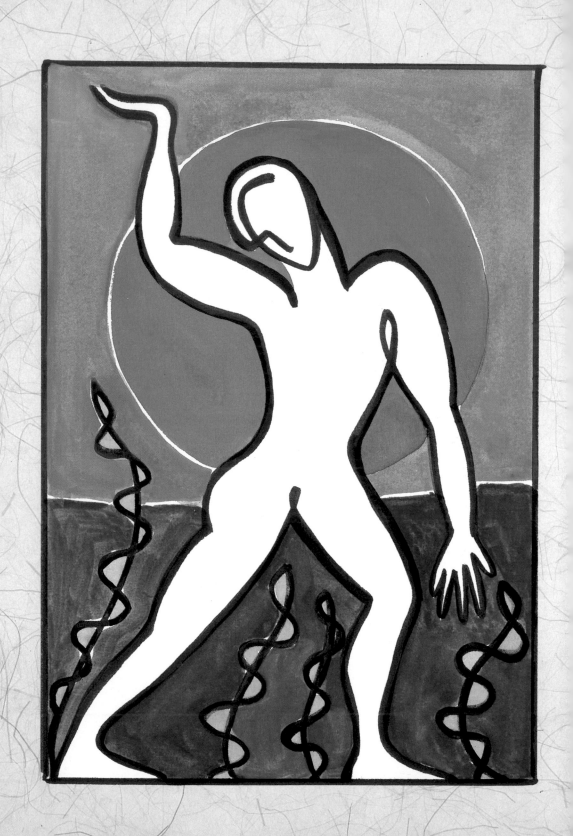

PART ONE

Heaven, Earth, and Human Beings

LEARNING THE BASICS

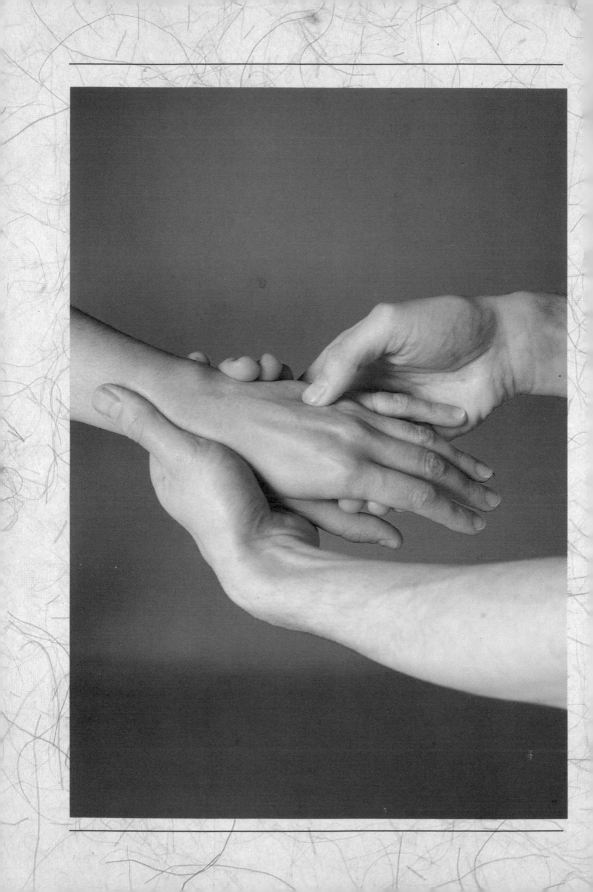

CHAPTER ONE

The Oriental Tradition

The traditional Oriental view of health takes wholeness as its starting point. It recognizes the universe as an energy field and all it contains as manifestations of energy in different patterns. Though infinitely varied, everything in the universe is connected; people are an intimate part of their environment and depend on it as much as they influence it. The primary tenet of Oriental medicine is to live in accord with nature, rather than trying to adapt nature to the needs of people.

Oriental medicine is based on observation of people and their response to the environment over thousands of years. Without the anatomical knowledge made available much later, Oriental theory established its own framework to explain how the body works and to explain natural phenomena (see Yin and Yang, pp. 18-23). The focus of attention is on how to maintain harmony within the body and with the outside world.

The Chinese observed the influence of the natural world and linked people's tendencies to particular types of ailment to the characteristics of the natural world (see The Five Elements, pp. 23-5). The emotions and lifestyle were also acknowledged as contributory factors in health and disease. To stay healthy, a person must continually adapt to the changes going on, both inside the body and out. If these adaptations are not made, illness manifests as disharmony within the body. Universal energy, called Ki, flows within the body forming a matrix that links the vital Organs with all the other parts. In treatment the emphasis is on restoring harmony to the Ki in the body. The physician's task is twofold: to interpret the cause, then to advise on appropriate lifestyle adjustments and to find a means of restoring the functions of the body.

Yin and Yang

Yin and Yang are concepts that are central to the unique viewpoint of traditional philosophy, science, and culture in China and Japan. Established from the observation of nature and society, they came to form the basis of traditional Chinese medicine, which then spread to Japan. Understanding the role of Yin and Yang is essential in learning about shiatsu: it forms the basis for all diagnosis and treatment.

Yin–Yang theory was first elaborated in the ancient and famous Chinese book of divination, *The Book of Changes* (I Ching), which dates in its earliest form to the 2nd millennium BC. It was well established by the time of Confucius, who added his commentaries in the 5th century BC. In this book Yang was represented by a continuous or "firm" line ▬▬ conveying direction and movement, and Yin by a broken or "yielding" line ▬ ▬ suggesting space and stillness. These lines were grouped in eight combinations of three, symbolizing all the basic permutations of natural forces and phenomena. Among these, three Yang lines grouped together ☰ represented "Heaven", the Yang archetype of the creative, active principle. Three Yin lines ☷ represented "Earth", the receptive or passive principle. Yang was regarded as masculine and Yin as feminine, and all life was seen as being dependent on their harmonious interaction. Light, warmth, and the passage of time were associated with the sun and its movement through Heaven; Earth offered material nourishment – food from the fields, shelter, and rest. The changing seasons and the repeating cycle of nights and days were deemed to be natural indications of the interrelatedness of Yin and Yang.

Unlike the idea of opposites inherited by Western culture from early Greek philosophy, the opposing qualities of Yin and Yang are seen as complementary and interdependent. They both create and control each other. When Yin declines, Yang expands, and vice versa, but there are no absolutes. Nothing can be wholly Yin or wholly Yang. Each contains the seed of the other: Yang will change into Yin; Yin into Yang.

Because everything has Yin and Yang characteristics to varying degrees, things can only be Yin or Yang

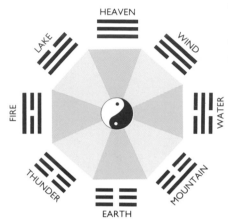

The 8 trigrams of the I Ching

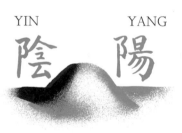

The Chinese characters for Yin and Yang mean, literally, the shady side and the sunny side of a hill, respectively. The hill represents existence, the "ground" in and around which Yin and Yang are in constant but ever-changing interplay.
Alone, Yin and Yang have no meaning. They cannot be separated either from each other or from existence itself.

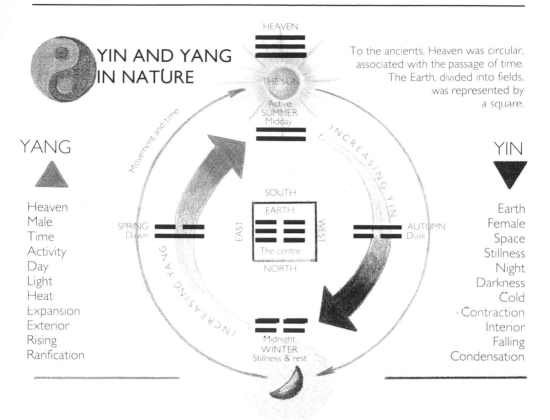

YIN AND YANG IN NATURE

HEAVEN

To the ancients, Heaven was circular, associated with the passage of time. The Earth, divided into fields, was represented by a square.

THE SUN

Active SUMMER Midday

INCREASING YIN

Movement and time

YANG

Heaven
Male
Time
Activity
Day
Light
Heat
Expansion
Exterior
Rising
Rarification

YIN

Earth
Female
Space
Stillness
Night
Darkness
Cold
· Contraction
Interior
Falling
Condensation

SPRING Dawn

EAST

SOUTH
EARTH
The centre
NORTH

WEST

AUTUMN Dusk

INCREASING YANG

Midnight WINTER Stillness & rest

---

relative to each other. Relative to the sun, the moon is Yin (cold, dense), but even the pale and watery moonlight is Yang relative to the surrounding night, and the shadowy caves and hollows where no light reaches.

The Tao

According to Lao Tzu (6th century BC) everything in the universe arose from the "Great Ultimate Source", or Tai Chi, represented by the famous symbol ☯. Beyond this was only emptiness, Wu Chi, represented as an empty circle ◯. The light and dark segments indicate the inherent duality in all things, as well as the interaction of Yin and Yang — the dynamic out of which life and all phenomena arise and continue to move and change. The law governing all these transformations was called the "Tao", meaning the "Way" of nature.

Ki

The Oriental view of life, nature, and the body is firmly founded on the notion of a vital force, or energy, which can be compared with the prana of Indian yogic philosophy. Its significance is so great in Oriental thinking, and its meaning so full of breadth and subtlety, that it is best to use the untranslated word "Ki" in the same way as we have become accustomed to use the Chinese words Yin and Yang.

Energy and matter

Ki arises from the interaction of Yin and Yang, and is the primary substance of the universe. This profoundly elegant understanding has existed in Eastern cultures for thousands of years. So it is said that all things are formed from Ki and that every different thing is determined or characterized by its Ki. Ki encompasses both the material and the non-material. In its "purer" form it is subtle and rarefied; it is "substance with no form". It is more Yang. Matter, on the other hand, is a condensed, "slowed-down" form of Ki. This is more Yin. It may seem paradoxical that Ki should exist as both matter and non-matter, but you may understand it more easily in terms of transformation and change.

Take the simple example of water boiling in a pot, transforming into steam, then condensing into droplets. Water is a more Yin state, steam is more Yang. The heat of the fire needed to boil water is intensely Yang (active), transforming the water into an expanded, Yang form. Coldness – relatively Yin – causes the condensation into droplets that collect on cooler surfaces or fall to earth. The most Yin form of water is ice. Ki is manifest in both the transformation and the substance: Yin Ki (of water) transforming into Yang Ki (steam) and then back into water. The paradox is contained. Matter and its changing state are characterized by its Ki. The universe, in its state of flux, sees the constant interplay of Yin and Yang, matter and non-matter.

Yin, Yang, and Ki in the body

The body depends on Ki, Blood and other essential substances, which change, flow, and circulate, and so are more Yang than the structural elements of the body. But here, too, Yin and Yang are at play together. Within the body Ki circulates in Channels, often called Meridians, which have no material form. Ki, similarly, has no physical structure and is, therefore, relatively Yang. It is the transforming power of the inner organs and is associated with activity, protection, and warmth. Traditionally, Ki is subdivided into many types according to its role in the body.

Blood is a liquid or materialized form of Ki. Its qualities are accordingly relatively Yin. Blood nourishes and supports the physical growth and renewal of body tissues and organs. It circulates in the blood vessels and is considered to have cooling and soothing properties.

Ki and Blood support and complement each

Human Being results from the Ki of Heaven and Earth. The union of the Ki of Heaven and Earth is called Human Being. THE YELLOW EMPEROR'S CLASSIC OF INTERNAL MEDICINE (c.100BC)

When Ki condenses it can form Beings. Quote attributed to ZHU XI (12th century AD)

The Body Structure

Within the body, Yin and Yang influences are always at work. The roles of Yin and Yang within the body structure are summarized right.

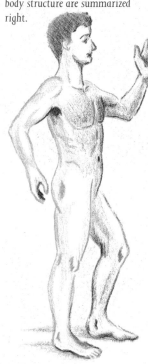

The living body has shape, structure, and weight. These are its Yin qualities. It is also active, warm, and responsive to its environment – attributes that are essentially Yang.

The head and the upper part of the body are more Yang; they are nearer Heaven. The feet and lower parts are more Yin; they are closer to the Earth.

The back and the exposed surfaces of the limbs are Yang. When we turn our backs against a cold wind, these are the strong, protective aspects we present to the outside.

The front and the protected inner aspects of the limbs are Yin. When we curl up in a defensive "armadillo" position, these are the soft, vulnerable inner surfaces we seek to protect.

The skin, the outermost layer of the physical body, and the muscles, the active body tissue that enables us to move, are both Yang.

The bones, the deepest, hardest, and most stable of the structural tissues, are Yin. So also are the internal organs, protected within the ribcage and the pelvic cavity. These are the deepest, most essential layer of our being.

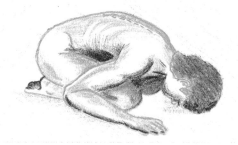

other. The Blood needs the Ki to keep it moving. The Ki needs the Blood to nourish the organs that generate it. Some Ki therefore flows with the Blood in the vessels and there is some Blood with the Ki in the Channels. "Ki is the leader of Blood; Blood is the mother of Ki." The *Yellow Emperor's Classic of Internal Medicine* (c.100BC)

Body Fluids

Body Fluids are the most Yin of the body substances. This general category includes the thick (most Yin) fluids that nourish the spinal cord and brain, and the thin (more Yang) lubricating fluids, including saliva, sweat, and tears, that moisten the skin and lubricate the openings of the sensory organs.

*The Yang Channels
flow downward, on
the backs of the
arms and legs.*

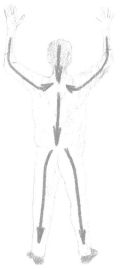

*The Yin Channels
flow up the front, inner
surfaces of the body.*

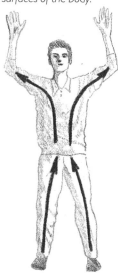

Mind and the spiritual attributes

The Chinese conceived the Spirit, or Mind, as a very rarefied body substance, the most Yang of all, associated with consciousness, intelligence, and will. The various aspects of the Spirit were thought to be housed in the Yin organs (see p. 23).

Organs, Channels, and the direction of Ki

Not only does Yin–Yang theory try to explain the relationship between the internal parts of the body, it also describes an "energetic" relationship between its inner and outer aspects – the vital organs and the surface. The supreme achievement of traditional Chinese medicine was perhaps that it perceived the inner organs as centres of transformation and distribution, which literally "organized" the entire body. This "organization" is mediated by the system of Channels that carries the Ki to all parts. It flows from within and circulates near the surface of the body. The internal condition of the body is reflected on the outside; work on the outside can affect the inside. In health, this is the body's regulating mechanism and allows us to adjust to the environment. In sickness, the mechanism breaks down, symptoms are produced on the outside. The ability to move Ki inside the body by giving treatment from the outside arises from the continuity of the energy network between inside and out. This is the "energetic" relationship.

The 12 main, or "Primary" Channels (see pp. 76–85) are dominated by the influence of either Heaven or Earth, producing accordingly either a downward flow from Heaven (Yang) or an upward flow from Earth (Yin). The Yang Channels are found on the back and on the outside surfaces of the arms and legs. They belong to the more superficial or "hollow" Organs of the digestive tract, principally the Stomach, Large and Small Intestines, Bladder, and Gall Bladder. Yang Organs are concerned with the processing of food and the elimination of waste; they are involved in the body's defensive functions and they are often implicated in the early or acute stages of illness. The Yin Channels are located on the front of the body and the inner surfaces of the limbs. They belong to the deep, "solid" Organs – the Lungs, Spleen, Heart, Kidneys, and Liver. The role of the

Yin Organs is the transformation, storage, and distribution of Ki and Blood and they are most affected in long-standing illness or weakness. The Yin and Yang Organs complement each other: each Yin Organ is paired with a Yang Organ in a reciprocal relationship (see pp. 79–80).

The Five Elements

The theory of Yin and Yang was not the only way by which the ancient Chinese interpreted the world. Early in the 1st millennium BC another system began to emerge in which all phenomena were seen as one of five manifestations resulting from transformations of Ki. These were known as the Five Elements, Five Transformations, or Five Phases, and were symbolically described as Water, Fire, Wood, Metal, and Earth. The *Shang Shu*, a text from this period, describes their qualities: "That which soaks and descends (Water) is salty, that which blazes upwards (Fire) is bitter, that which can be bent and straightened (Wood) is sour, that which can be moulded and become hard (Metal) is pungent, that which permits sowing and reaping (Earth) is sweet." The Five Elements were also associated with the seasons, colours, sounds, mythical animals, grains, and many other things and events. So a system of correspondences gradually developed to build up a picture of the connections in the natural world (see the chart on page 25).

Around the 4th century BC, a time of turmoil and change in China, the search for order and meaning in the relationship between people and their environment led to the expansion of Five Element theory. Things were more than just categorized; their capacity to change, interact, and transform into each other was recognized and described in various ways.

The early physicians based their understanding of the cause and development of illness on the interrelating patterns of the Five Elements (see p. 24). Each Organ was either nourished or controlled by one of the others. Disease could progress from one Organ to another through lack of nourishment, "over-control", or its opposite, "insult". Treatment of a deficient or malfunctioning Organ was often given by strengthening

Development of Five Element theory

The Five Elements soon became integrated into Yin–Yang theory and the two were developed together by a philosophical school called the Naturalists. An early model of the Five Element relationships is reminiscent of the Yin–Yang diagram (see right and p. 19). This early model shows the important balance between Water and Fire, with Water representing downward movement, stillness, and rest, but full of potential power, and Fire representing upward movement and climax of activity. The complementary yet opposing tendencies, Wood and Metal, represented expansion or outward movement and contraction or inward movement respectively. Earth was seen as a moderating influence on the season, having no season of its own. It is like a pivot or reference point for change.

Later, other arrangements were developed in which Earth occupied a position equal to the other Elements. Two in particular became established for representing natural order in the world; both the way in which things progress and support each other, called the generating sequence (see right), and the way in which they restrain or limit each other, called the controlling sequence (see far right).

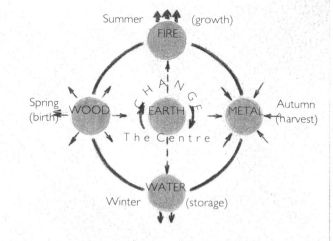

Early Yin–Yang model representing the Five Elements.

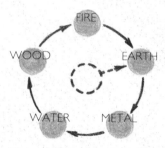

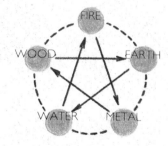

Generating sequence

Wood fuels Fire; Fire's ashes enrich the Earth; Metal is found in the Earth; Water condenses on Metal; and Water feeds Wood.

Controlling sequence

Wood (plant matter) stabilizes the Earth; Earth contains Water within its banks; Water controls Fire; Fire melts Metal and Metal (tools) cuts Wood.

the Organ preceding it in the sequence known as the "generating sequence" (see above).

The usefulness of this system extends beyond the portrayal of harmonious interaction since it can also predict or interpret the effects of disharmony, when things get "out of phase" and inevitably balance is lost. For example, if Fire is weak the effect of Water will be more than mere control, threatening to extinguish it altogether. This is known as over-acting of one Element

NATURE	Wood	Fire	Earth	Metal	Water
Directions	East	South	Centre	West	North
Seasons	Spring	Summer	Transition	Autumn	Winter
Climates	Wind	Heat	Dampness	Dryness	Cold
Cyclic Stages	Birth	Growth	Ripening	Harvest	Storing
Colours	Green	Red	Yellow	White	Black/Blue
Flavours	Sour	Bitter	Sweet	Pungent	Salty
HUMAN BODY					
Yin Organs	Liver	Heart	Spleen	Lungs	Kidneys
Yang Organs	Gall Bladder	Small Intestine	Stomach	Large Intestine	Bladder
Sense Organs	Eyes	Tongue	Mouth	Nose	Ears
Senses	Sight	Speech	Taste	Smell	Hearing
Body Tissues	Ligaments & Tendons	Blood Vessels	Muscles (Flesh)	Skin	Bones
Manifestation	Nails	Face (Complexion)	Lips	Body Hair	Head Hair
Fluids	Tears	Sweat	Saliva	Mucus	Urine
Sounds	Shouting	Laughing	Singing	Weeping	Groaning
Emotions	Anger	Joy	Pensiveness/ Worry	Grief	Fear
Spiritual Aspects	Ethereal Soul	Mind	Intellect	Corporeal Soul	Will

When the Emperor Huang Ti questioned his physician Ch'i Po, he answered: "The East creates the wind, wind creates the wood; wood creates the sour flavour. The sour flavour strengthens the Liver, the Liver nourishes the tendons, the tendons strengthen the Heart and the Liver governs the eyes. The eyes see the darkness and mystery of Heaven and they discover the Tao, the Right Way among Mankind. Anger is injurious to the Liver, but pensiveness counteracts anger. Wind is injurious to the tendons but heat and dryness counteract the wind. The sour flavour can injure the tendons but the pungent flavour counteracts the sour flavour." THE YELLOW EMPEROR'S CLASSIC OF INTERNAL MEDICINE (c.100BC)

on another. Similarly, if Water is deficient then Fire can vaporize it, thus overcoming the Element that usually controls it. This reversal of the controlling sequence is called counteracting, or "insulting".

The development of medicine progressed with the extension of the Five Element theory to include the body's major organs, the sensory organs and body tissues, the human emotions, and subtle spiritual qualities. Combined with external factors, such as season, climate, foods, and so on (see pp. 154–165), the whole picture of correspondences provided a reference for diagnosis and healing. A table of the traditional Five Element correspondences is given above.

As Chinese medicine developed through the centuries, the Five Elements were accorded greater or lesser importance, but their usefulness is still widely recognized today as a general system of medical reference. The Five Element system is particularly well regarded in Japan and the practice of shiatsu is greatly enhanced by a knowledge of this traditional approach.

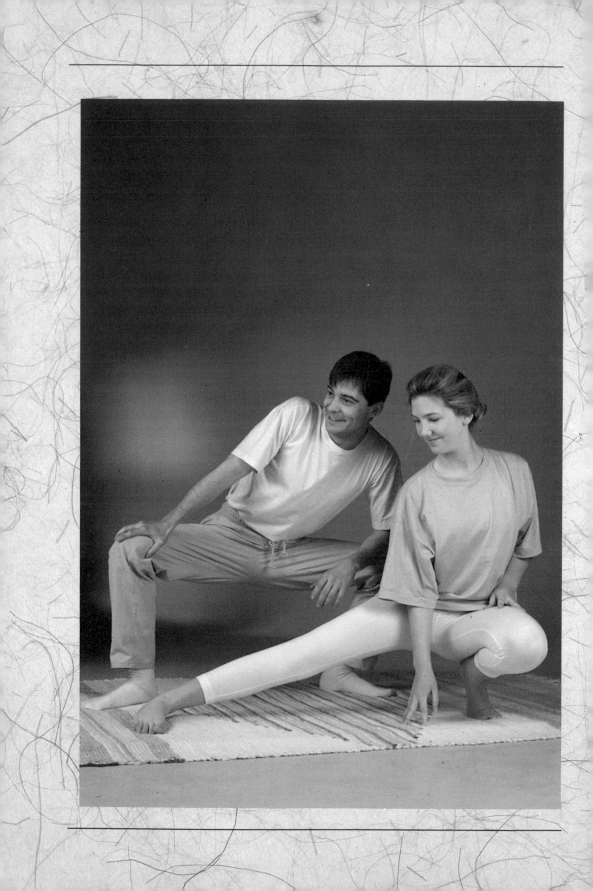

CHAPTER TWO

Your Own Wellbeing

To heal others, begin with yourself. Giving shiatsu to your friends will not be easy if you are tired, frustrated, weak, or sick. Whatever your constitution, good health springs from maintaining a balance in your diet, exercise, rest, security, level of challenge, and so on. Finding this balance means looking after yourself physically, mentally, and emotionally, and taking responsibility for your own condition. This may not be easy: self-discovery is a lifetime's work. Acknowledge your weaknesses as well as your strengths; learn to recognize when you need help and ask for it; accept as well as give. All these are important steps on the way to gaining an inner harmony that will bring healing qualities to your work.

Shiatsu helps you on this path. As a way to health it is as enjoyable to give as to receive, and the practice of shiatsu develops not only your physical fitness but your intuition and understanding as well. This chapter presents traditional healing exercises for the practitioner and receiver, which integrate Body, Breath, and Mind, and harmonize Yin and Yang. You will gain these subtle internal benefits through grounding exercises (see pp. 28-35), breathing exercises (see pp. 39-41), and sometimes through the use of visualization or concentration (see pp. 40-1). These exercises are central to the practice of shiatsu, for beginners as well as the more accomplished.

Most shiatsu sessions take place on the floor. The grounding exercises at the beginning of this chapter are designed to give you a "feel" for the ground and to develop the flexibility and strength to enable you to work at floor level for extended periods. Exercises to allow you to obtain the same level of flexibility and strength in your fingers, your basic tools in shiatsu, follow the floor positions (see pp. 36-7).

Grounding

To practise shiatsu well, you must learn what it means to be in touch with the ground and feel its effect on the physical body. Gravity, the "Earth-Force", conditions our total experience. From infancy we have to contend with it. Our muscular system is engaged from the outset in the effort of raising up the head, wriggling, crawling, and eventually learning to stand and walk. This process develops the secondary curves of the spine – in the neck and lumbar region – and influences our posture, grace, and balance from an early age.

Begin with some exercises on the floor to enhance your connection with the ground and remove the tensions produced by standing upright (see pp. 28–35). The exercises on all fours (see pp. 30–1) will loosen and balance the curves of your spine and benefit your nervous system. Grounding exercises increase your awareness of your body weight. They will teach you to use the ground for support: to get down and make friends with the floor; to crawl, kneel, or squat, and move comfortably on all fours. We need to feel and imbue our bodies with this feeling of support in order to convey it in our work with others.

Practice time

Create your own routine from the exercises described on the following pages. Do the exercises at any convenient time, not necessarily before giving shiatsu. You need only practise for 10–30 minutes at a time, but as your stamina improves you may want to work for longer. Practise every day if you want to, but three or four times a week is still useful. Your body will tell you what your needs and limitations are if you listen.

Comfort and safety

When giving shiatsu or practising the preparatory exercises that follow you should wear loose, comfortable clothes to allow full freedom of movement. Garments made from natural fibres help prevent over-heating. Put on a sweater after exercising to prevent you from getting chilled. Avoid draughts.

Be sensible about these exercises. Don't push or strain. Work into any stiffness and resistance gradually. Look after yourself. The exercises are designed to enhance your power as a healer.

Bowing

Bowing is used both as a social and religious gesture among Eastern peoples. It signifies respect and service to another person or "higher being". In Japan the practice of bowing has many nuances, which help to smooth the passage of daily life. It is also an essential part of martial arts practice for students, teachers, and opponents. Bowing is not only symbolic. As with many rituals, there is a practical purpose to it. It has a very calming, purifying, and focusing effect on the body and mind and makes an appropriate starting point for your exercises on the floor.

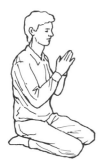

Position 1

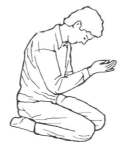

Position 2

Kneel comfortably on the floor, or on a cushion. Bring your palms together at chest level, arms slightly extended (position 1). Relax, exhale, and then inhaling deeply, imagine "Heaven's Energy" flowing down through your hands or the top of your head as you fill your lungs.

Exhale easily and slowly, dipping your head a little while opening your hands in symbolic offering to the "Heaven Force" (position 2). Inhale and return to the starting position.

Now exhale deeply and fold forward at the hips. Separate your hands to place them, palms down, on the floor. Relax completely, chest on knees. Let your forehead touch the ground or "Earth" (position 3). Remain quiet and still, momentarily giving up all your thoughts. Allow your next inhalation to fill your body and, thinking of life breathing into you, return naturally to the upright position.

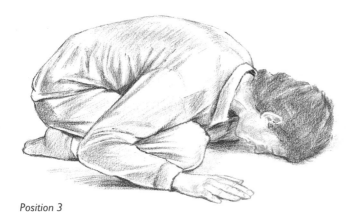

Position 3

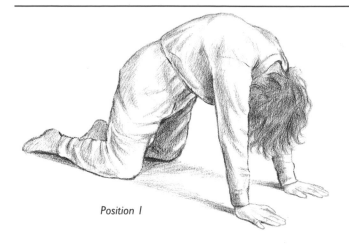

Position 1

ON ALL FOURS

This series of exercises, based on the "dog postures" of yoga, will help to counteract any stiffness in your spine by first stretching it, then relaxing it. It allows you to feel the physical weight of your chest and belly, which should literally hang from your spine, supported at each end by your arms and legs. Each exercise begins from a comfortable "all-fours" position with your arms and thighs at right angles to the ground.

Position 2

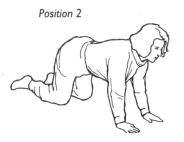

Relax on all fours. Now let your head drop and, inhaling, arch your spine high (position 1). Stretch your back in the arched position, pause, then on a long, easy out breath let your back relax right down, so your spine hangs naturally (position 2). Breathe easily for a few moments and repeat.

Start in the "all fours" position. Tuck in your toes, then lift yourself off your knees, stretch your legs back, and raise your buttocks toward the sky. Press back from your hands, relaxing your head, and let your chest move toward your legs to narrow the inverted "V" shape (position 1). Stretch your knees and lower your heels. They need not touch the floor. Exhale as you move into and out of this position. Breathe easily as you hold it for a few moments.

Position 2

Exhale and lower your hips to the floor, supporting the front of your body on your hands. Now raise and tighten your knees, stretching your legs, toes flat. Look up to the sky, but don't strain your head back (position 2). Breathe easily, holding the position for just a few moments.

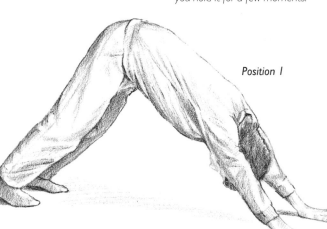

Position 1

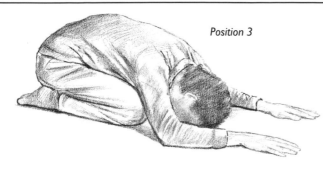

Position 3

Relax by sinking on to your haunches, folding at the hips. Let your chest rest on your thighs, and your head touch the ground. Place your arms forward (position 3) or alongside your legs. Breathe into your belly. This "pose of the child" is rejuvenating and relaxing.

Shifting the weight

This exercise develops a fluidity of movement between hips, spine, and shoulder joints, and strength and flexibility in the wrists. It also familiarizes you with the feeling of shifting your centre of gravity to transfer weight through your limbs in your shiatsu sessions.

Still on all fours, relax your spine and belly and begin slow, clockwise movements. Bring your body weight forward on to your left then right hand, then back into your right and left hips. Make several circles, then reverse the direction.

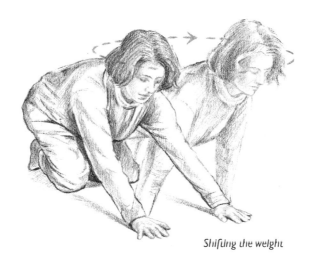

Shifting the weight

Belly consciousness

Conditioning often encourages us to hold in our stomach muscles either for the sake of appearance or to distance our thoughts and feelings from our lower parts. But we should rather be like the animals. Let your spine relax and your belly hang down. Then energy and blood will circulate naturally in your abdomen and you will develop a strong centre. In Japan the belly is known as the "Hara" (see Chapter 3). Holding your belly in is a sign of tension. Whenever you find yourself doing it, breathe out, relax, and let go.

The natural crawl

Crawling is something many of us have not done for years. Even in childhood, many of us were encouraged too quickly through this important stage, which is now thought to influence the development of intelligence. Children are praised for each early step and in this manner proceed through schooling and adult, career-oriented lives favouring the intellect and "higher" things, weakening their relationship with the ground at each stage. We must "stand on our own two feet", become "upright citizens", "walk tall", "make it to the top", and so on. Unfortunately

we may have to stiffen up to meet these expectations. So it can be a relief to get down and practise crawling again.

Begin slowly from the previous exercise. You know how to do it! Crawl naturally around the room, noticing how you keep your balance on three limbs as you raise and move the fourth one. If you crawl very slowly, even stop and move backward, you will discover something very important for shiatsu — the ability to increase or reduce your weight through one limb just by moving from your centre.

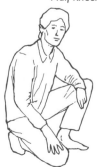

Kneeling in seiza

SITTING AND SQUATTING

For people in much of the world, sitting and squatting on the ground are familiar positions. Work in the fields, cooking, eating, craftwork, and ceremonial activities involve continual squatting, bending, and kneeling. Our more sedentary life-style has made these positions alien and difficult. Sitting at desks and working with modern appliances and machines is the cause of many problems of the back, abdomen, and pelvis. Practise kneeling and squatting — they are good for you.

The seiza posture

Seiza is the natural sitting position for the Japanese in daily life, which is traditionally organized at floor level. This sitting position also has formal connotations. Japanese people sit in seiza before performing martial arts, during the tea ceremony, or for Zen meditation where the object is just to sit. It provides a stable base and is easy to return to, and move from. When sitting still, the feet act like a cushion that lifts the back and helps keep the spine straight. For these reasons many prefer it to the cross-legged position of other traditional cultures. It is the best position for beginning shiatsu because other kneeling or squatting postures flow naturally from it.

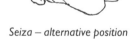

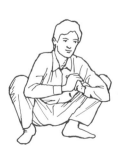

Seiza — alternative position

Kneel with your back relaxed but straight, buttocks resting on your heels, feet together (see above left), or between your spread heels, toes pointing inward. The variation (see left) with the toes tucked up and under gives you support, a rest, and makes a change. If your knees are stiff practise kneeling on a cushion or rolled blanket.

Half-kneeling position   Toe-raised squat   Flat-foot squat

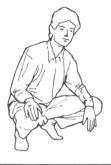

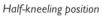

These squatting positions are simple ways to increase or maintain your flexibility. Any style is beneficial: use them while you chat to friends or watch television.

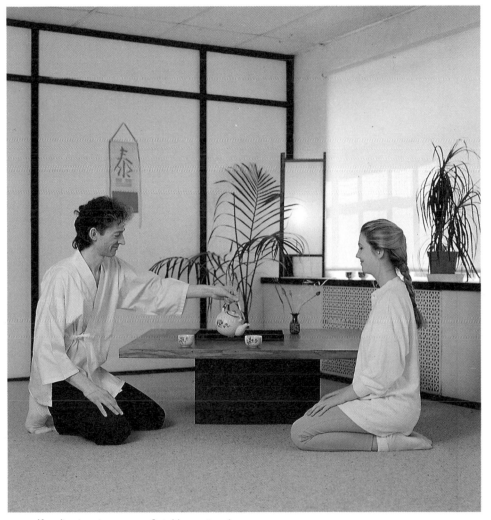

Kneeling in seiza – a comfortable way to relax.

Low standing exercises

We feel understandably protective of the body's lower regions, but many of us become tense and "closed-off" from our lower selves. Sitting with the thighs crossed demonstrates this need for protection. Such habits do nothing for the posture or circulation. The exercises on this page open the groin and encourage blood to flow to the organs and muscles of the lower abdomen and pelvic floor. However, these low stretches are strenuous and demanding. Do them carefully and follow the directions given. Only move on to the more demanding positions shown on p. 35 when you are fully comfortable in those shown below.

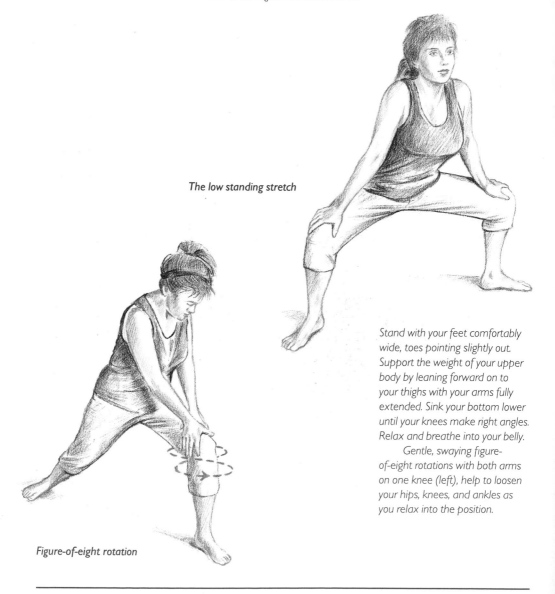

The low standing stretch

Figure-of-eight rotation

Stand with your feet comfortably wide, toes pointing slightly out. Support the weight of your upper body by leaning forward on to your thighs with your arms fully extended. Sink your bottom lower until your knees make right angles. Relax and breathe into your belly.

Gentle, swaying figure-of-eight rotations with both arms on one knee (left), help to loosen your hips, knees, and ankles as you relax into the position.

From the low standing stretch, turn your right foot out, pivoting on the heel, and the left heel out, pivoting on the ball of your left foot. Now turn to face right, bring your left hand over and lean with both arms on your thigh. Keep your trunk upright, open your chest, and lift your spine; gaze forward and breathe fully. Tighten your back knee gently and look up (see right). Hold for a few seconds, then relax, turn through the centre, and repeat on the other side.

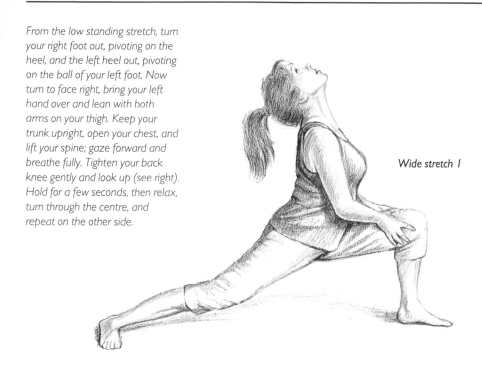

Wide stretch 1

Wide stretch 2

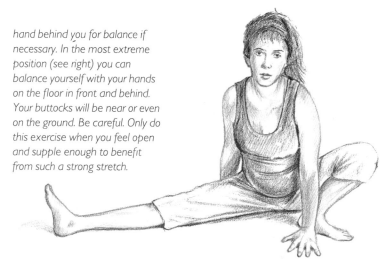

From the low standing stretch move your body weight over to one side and lean one hand or arm on your folded thigh for support. Extend your other leg, gradually edging your foot out. Sink down, lean forward and place one or both hands on the floor to steady yourself. Turn the toes of your extended foot skyward, rolling on to your heel. The folded leg, carrying most of your weight, may feel more secure with the heel raised at first, but gradually practise lowering it. Move one hand behind you for balance if necessary. In the most extreme position (see right) you can balance yourself with your hands on the floor in front and behind. Your buttocks will be near or even on the ground. Be careful. Only do this exercise when you feel open and supple enough to benefit from such a strong stretch.

Hand exercises

Our fingers, hands, and wrists are our main tools in shiatsu. Their strength and flexibility are particularly important. The exercises below, familiar to musicians, sportspeople, and masseurs alike, can be practised in any way: as part of a complete body routine; as a sequence on their own; or singly at any time. Try them while waiting for a bus or train and ignore strange looks from passers-by!

Keep your mind on your posture even while concentrating on your hands. Relax your shoulders and try not to frown, grit your teeth, or hold your breath. Ease up and relax. Give your hands a good shake now and then, between exercises. Remember, they hold tension just as much as any other part of the body.

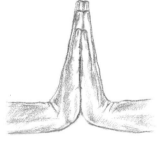

Stretching the wrists

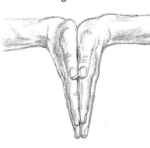

Sitting comfortably, bring your palms together close to your chest, fingers pointing upward. Press your hands together and push your wrists down to stretch them (top left). Relax, and repeat once or twice. Then turn your hands to point down and stretch by pushing the wrists upward (bottom left). Relax your shoulders. Next, interlock your fingers, turn your hands out, and stretch your fingers, palms, and wrists by extending your arms (right).

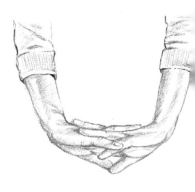

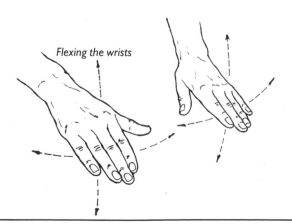

Flexing the wrists

Move your wrists from side to side, up and down, then flip them over, palms facing up (supination), and flip them back, palms down (pronation). Then move your hands in any of these ways, in the same or opposite directions, repeating them first slowly, then quickly. Keep your arms relaxed.

Working on the fingers

Fingers are used in special ways in the practice of shiatsu. They need strength, flexibility, and a relaxed sensitivity. You need to lean your weight through the fingers and thumbs in most shiatsu techniques, rather than simply press with the fingers. Often, too, you use the fingers to provide stability while leaning through the thumbs. Even more important, the fingers are for feeling. They will tell you much about the physical and "energetic" condition of the people you work with.

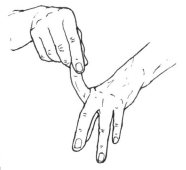

Loosening the fingers

Extend your fingers one at a time, then grasp each one in turn by the tip, and stretch it back (see left). Hold it for a moment. Then rotate or "stir" each finger in turn around the knuckle joint.

To increase the reach of your fingers, insert your fist between each of the fingers of your other hand (see left). Open the space between your thumb and first finger by pressing them together, as shown (see right).

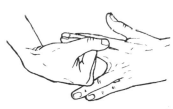
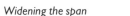

Widening the span

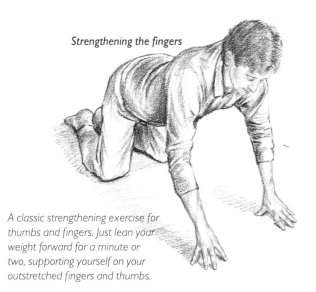

Stretching the fingers

Hold your hands in front of you, and slowly clench your fists as though crushing rocks into powder. Then open them slowly as though against enormous pressure. Repeat a few times. Then open and close your fists lightly and rapidly as a contrast. Ask yourself: did you stop breathing, pull faces, clench your teeth, or tighten your shoulders? Relax, it will come.

Strengthening the fingers

A classic strengthening exercise for thumbs and fingers. Just lean your weight forward for a minute or two, supporting yourself on your outstretched fingers and thumbs.

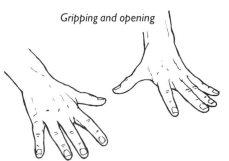

Gripping and opening

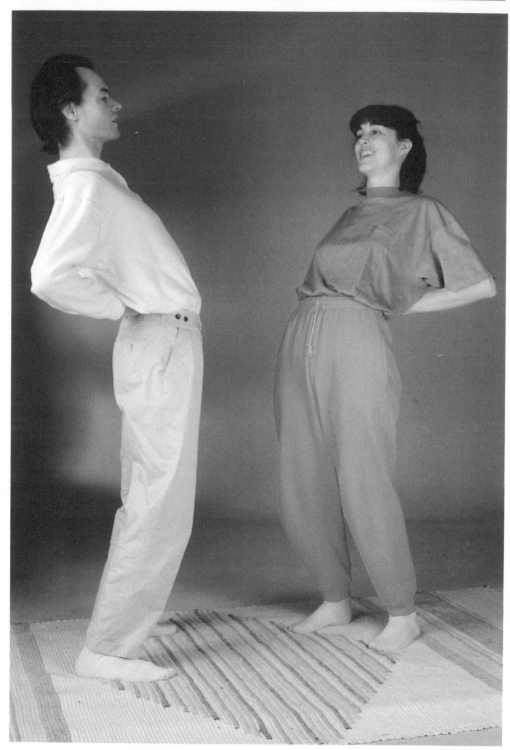

The bow posture

Breathing

Tension, anxiety, and shock restrict the movement of the diaphragm and rib muscles and can inhibit the respiratory mechanism. Consequent shallow breathing limits your energy. The exercises that follow counteract this restriction and will enable you to work more strongly with your breath, increasing the power of your movements. All these exercises begin from a standing position. With your feet firmly planted on the "Earth" you can reach up into "Heaven's Realm", which is traditionally associated with Ki in Oriental medicine. The Lungs circulate this vital energy through the Channels to all parts of the body, through the diaphragm and into the belly, or Hara, where it is concentrated at the vital centre known in Japan as the "Tanden" This is the equivalent of the centre of gravity in the physical body. The energies of Heaven and Earth unite here to bring power, harmony, and spontaneity to our actions.

The forward bend

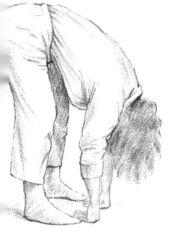

This is a relaxing position. Make no effort other than to breathe deeply into your Hara. Let your head hang from your neck and your arms hang loosely from your shoulders. Bend your knees slightly. Relax further and sink lower with each exhalation. Keep your weight evenly distributed over your heels and toes. Slowly uncurl when you are ready.

The bow

The bow posture (see p. 38) stretches open the chest and diaphragm. Stand firmly, feet apart, knees slightly bent, and support your back by placing your fists or palms wherever feels most comfortable. Bend backward from your hips, making a smooth curve with your back — like a bow. Keep your gaze straight ahead: looking upward distracts and uproots you. Inhale and exhale deeply, opening your chest, diaphragm, and belly. Your lower back and your shoulders will tend to tighten up; try to relax them and keep your shoulders down. After a minute or so, straighten up gently and move slowly into the full forward bend (see above left). The two exercises are complementary and will increase your energy levels.

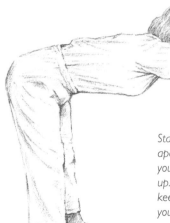

The half bend

Stand with feet a shoulder-width apart, knees relaxed. Slowly raise your arms above your head. Look up. Point your fingers inward and keep your elbows curved, so that your arms form a circle around your head. Then breathe out smoothly and, keeping your legs straight but not locked tight, fold at the hips until your trunk is horizontal, with your arms still extended in front (see above). Pause, breathe smoothly, and look out between your hands. Lift and open your chest. After a few breaths, exhale and continue down into a forward bend. Relax.

1

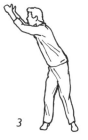

2

3

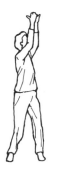

4

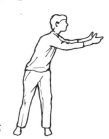

5

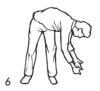

6

Carrying the circle

From the forward bend (position 1) with your elbows relaxed and slightly bent, imagine that your arms are encircling a ball of energy, which is recharged every time you breathe in. Think of the Earth giving your feet support, or uplift. This will help to keep your feet firmly planted, giving you a stable base for movement.

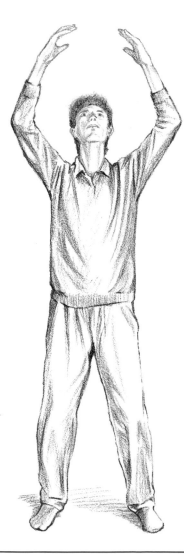

Exhale gently and turn your trunk to the right, leaning your weight over your right foot (2). Breathe in slowly and deeply and raise your body (3), lifting your circle out and up, until you are upright, gazing skyward between your fingers (see left). Exhale and turn your body slowly to face left (4). Inhale, and, on a long exhalation, fold at the hips, weight over your left foot, and carry the circle lightly down, extending your arms and body to the left (5 and 6). Inhale again at the bottom (1). Complete 2 or 3 circles in each direction, finishing in the forward bend (1). Release your arms and uncurl into the upright position.

Unifying the mind, body, and breath

As you learn to coordinate your breath and your body movement, you will find that you can work slowly, smoothly, and with the minimum of effort. This is one of the basic principles of the Chinese exercise systems known as Tao Yin and Chi Kung: it is movement from a relaxed state of mind. The mind, remaining calm, centred, and detached, directs the Ki, which influences the physical attributes of the body. The mind harmonizes the breath with the body movement, and this harmony is the path to inner health. The Chi Kung tradition teaches that "The Mind controls the Ki, Ki moves but the Mind does not move." The simplest method used in Chi Kung to achieve this stillness of mind is to listen to the sound of your breathing, to concentrate on your body movements as you do them, and to gaze toward the far horizon (whether you are inside or outside), without attaching your mind to external objects.

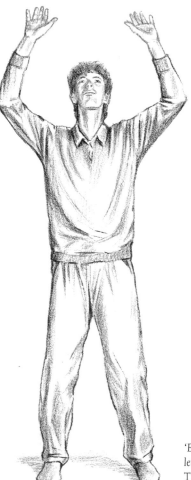

Stand on the Earth, support the Sky

From the outside this posture is static, but as you concentrate on the supportive Ki of the Earth you will feel the internal dynamic of the exercise. Allow this quality to move right through you, adding power to your arms in supporting the Sky.

Raise your arms slowly on an inhalation and turn your palms skyward so that they are pressing gently upward (see right). Alternatively you can move straight into this exercise from the highest position in "Carrying the circle" (see p. 40): just turn your wrists to move your hands into position. Relax your elbows and knees, bending them slightly.

Breathe in Heaven's Ki. As you exhale, direct it to your feet and palms. Support the Sky, without effort. After a while, let go. Lower your arms, and relax (see far right). Stand quietly, breathing calmly for a few minutes.

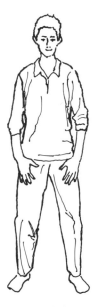

'Empty yourself of everything and let the mind be at peace.'
TAO TE CHING, LAO TZU

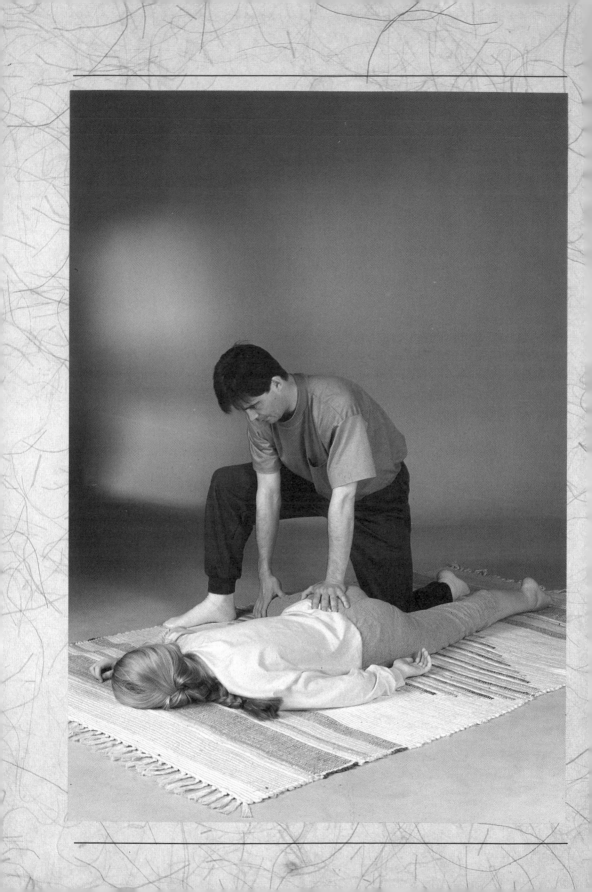

CHAPTER THREE

Principles and Techniques

Whatever our work, we need the best tools available. The better their quality and accuracy, the more pleasant the task, and the more effective the outcome. Shiatsu is enjoyable, interesting, and rewarding, but it is work nonetheless. Your "tools" are the parts of your body, mainly hands and fingers, and you are the instrument that coordinates them. This chapter will familiarize you with new ways of using your body - rather like a manual for adjusting a fine instrument. The I Ching (Book of Changes) tells us that perseverance brings success; it suggests that we take time and seek help on the way. Use this chapter often as a source of reference as you work through the book.

The special techniques and principles of shiatsu allow us to use the physical body effectively without strain or tiredness. The basic shiatsu techniques for giving pressure (see pp. 45-9) allow us to transmit Ki through the body to our partners. The stretches and rotations that follow (see pp. 50-1) open the Channels and loosen the joints, which improves the flow of Ki. By learning and practising the more advanced techniques explained in the last part of the chapter (see pp. 52-5) you can develop the subtle qualities that bring natural power and vitality to your shiatsu.

At a practical level remember you will need a few "accessories". First, the floor. Work on something firm but comfortable, a thick carpet or folded blanket is fine, but the traditional Japanese three-layer "futon" mattress is ideal for shiatsu. Use a flat pillow for your partner's head, a few cushions for ankles and knees, a quiet space if you can find one. That's all.

Tools and techniques

You can use almost every part of your body in your shiatsu practice. All shiatsu techniques involve leaning your body weight through your fingers, thumbs, palms, elbows, knees, or feet. Effective shiatsu depends on the way you apply pressure through these parts on to your partner. The illustrations on pages 44–9 demonstrate shiatsu techniques for applying pressure with each part of your body.

To palm, cover the area on your partner's body with your open hand. Lean your body weight through your palm. Then lean back to slide your hand a little further along, and lean again. Let it follow the shape of your partner's body. With practice you will learn to emphasize your pressure with different parts of your hand.

Palming the inner leg

Palming
Palming is one of the simplest and most commonly used shiatsu techniques. It means "leaning" or "holding" with the open palm. Palm pressure is gentle but firm; it is supportive, comforting, and tonifying — encouraging Ki to flow and restoring circulation to areas of underlying weakness. Use the palming technique to soothe away stiffness and defensive reactions in each part of the body before continuing your work with the thumbing technique (see facing page).

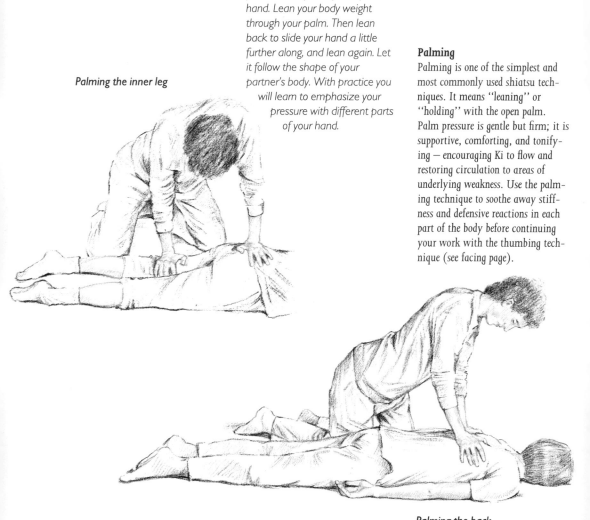

Palming the back

First principles of pressure

Teachers of the Zen style of shiatsu remind us to use body weight, not pressure. "Lean, don't press", they say, yet shiatsu is always described in terms of pressure. It is difficult to think of pressure that is not "pressing". To give good shiatsu you should lean and let your body weight work for you, rather than push or press. Masunaga described this as "penetrating pressure", which combined three elements of technique: perpendicular pressure, stationary pressure, and supporting pressure (see pp. 48–9). It has nothing to do with force of effort, it is something that allows the Ki of the giver and receiver to interact.

Listening to your partner

The best way to "listen" or tune yourself to your partner's Ki while applying pressure is to pay attention to their breathing – sometimes shallow, sometimes deeper, sometimes held, or released with a sigh. Relax and let yourself be taught by what you feel. Then you can move on.

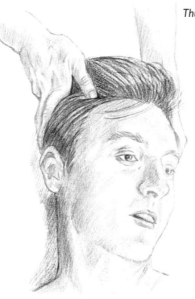

Thumbing

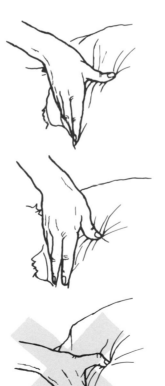

Thumbing

The thumb is more penetrating, precise, and generally more stimulating than the palm. It is the "finger" most commonly used in shiatsu. Always use the thumb extended: think of it as a direct continuation of the line of your arm. Do not bend the thumb at the first joint, or use the muscles of the thumb to press the point (see bottom left). Both detract from sensitivity and feeling, make you tired, and are likely to produce too weak or too strong a pressure, depending on your own strength.

Give pressure by leaning your weight through the thumb tip, a strong technique, or by holding the ball of the thumb rather more flat, which is milder. Steady the thumb by extending the fingers (see above). Never use it on its own. Note: always keep your nails short for your shiatsu sessions.

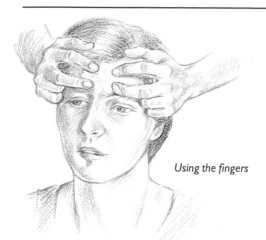

Using the fingers

The thumb and finger can be used together when two close points are treated at once, usually along either side of the body's mid line – on the head, the neck, the spine, or the sacral region. The thumb and finger are particularly useful when the other hand is being used for support, as shown below.

Use the fingers for delicate and precise work on the face. Each hand can work on either side of the mid line. Using both hands together (see above) gives a feeling of stability.

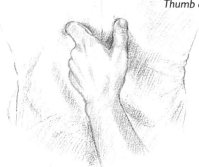

Thumb and finger

Thumb and knuckle

The "Dragon's Mouth" technique is particularly useful for work along the edge of the forearm. The fingers and thumb provide stability on either side of the arm; by a small forward-rolling motion of your wrist you apply precise pressure through the knuckle at the base of the forefinger.

This is a more robust alternative to the thumb and finger technique, especially if your fingers are long. It is suited to working down either side of the spine of a muscular back with one hand. Use the knuckle or middle section of the folded forefinger to match the pressure given by the ball of the thumb.

"Dragon's Mouth"

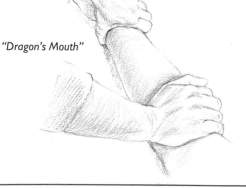

Using the elbows, knees, and feet

There are three reasons for using the elbows, knees, and feet. First, thumbs and fingers can get tired from the physical demands of shiatsu. Second, elbows, knees, and feet are suited to work on the stronger or more robust people and parts of the body. The third reason is that elbows and knees are excellent for working into stiff or painful muscles associated with tension. Using the elbow or knee in this way is known as "sedation technique". It enables you to penetrate the areas of blocked Ki in a "friendly" way, dispersing it and reducing pain. The heel of the hand can be used to similar effect.

Elbow technique is very versatile. It can be used on the shoulders, the back, buttocks, hips, thighs, lower legs, and sometimes even the arms.

The only foot techniques described in this book are specifically for working on the receiver's feet. They are safe, easy to practise and very pleasant to receive, and provide the giver with a welcome break from the ground.

Before you begin, use your fingers to feel the shape and condition of the area you are working on, then locate your elbow comfortably with their help. Hold your own arms open at the elbow and work with the flattened underside of the angle, not on the "points" (see right). Lean without pressing.

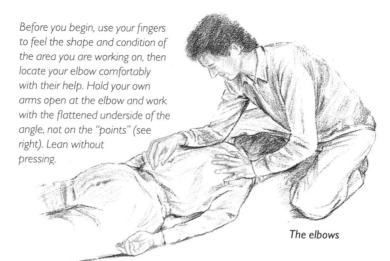

The elbows

Knee technique, used mainly on the legs, particularly the thighs, demands good balance and a relaxed body. Support yourself comfortably on all fours, hands in contact with the receiver. Then take more weight on to your hands and raise one knee into position, slowly transferring your weight on to that knee so the receiver experiences comfortable pressure.

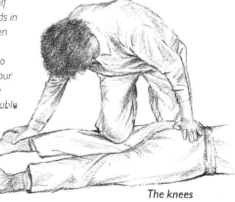

The knees

Standing on your partner's feet

Either stand with your own heels on your partner's feet (facing away from them), or use the balls of your feet (see right). Keep part of each foot in touch with the ground. Transfer your weight gradually on to their feet. Shift from foot to foot to find comfortable positions.

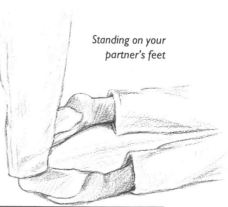

Leaning on a wall

Body leaning
By leaning your whole body (as shown on this and the facing page), you are using all three elements of penetrating pressure (see right). The exercises shown on these pages are designed to help you understand the difference between leaning and pressing (see p. 45).

You can experience secure leaning very easily. Pick a good wall and lean on it to your heart's content — and feel the support.

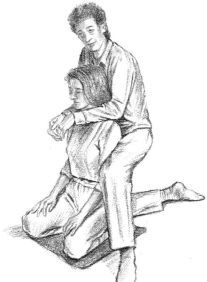

*Shoulder leaning
(alternative version)*

These simple shoulder-leaning techniques contain the three elements of penetrating pressure: perpendicular, stationary, and support pressure. Ask your partner to sit cross-legged on a cushion, or kneel as shown, firmly planted and secure. (see left and right)
*   Then relax your weight, leaning at right angles, on to your partner's shoulders. Be aware of the support that they, in turn, are giving you. Support your partner's back with your thigh or knee (see right). You should both be comfortable. Try leaning on your elbows on different parts of the shoulders (see left).*

PENETRATING PRESSURE
The elements of pressure outlined on page 45 are described in greater detail below.

Perpendicular pressure
Always keep a right angle between the direction of your pressure and your partner's body. This is the Yang component of penetrating pressure; the best way to contact the Ki — straight in.

Stationary pressure
Leaning your body weight without moving is a more passive, receptive, Yin aspect of shiatsu. When your hands are still you can tune into your partner's Ki. You need do nothing — the Ki will respond because its nature is to move. Any extra movements you make may obscure this response.

Supporting pressure
You are already familiar with the idea of the ground as our support (see pp. 28–32). Supporting pressure is both a technique in which we

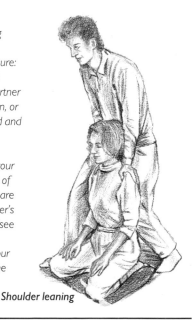

Shoulder leaning

support our partner, and a quality of touch that conveys care, consideration, and safety. It is another hidden, Yin, Earth-related aspect of good shiatsu.

The support hand

This provides a balance for the pressure being applied with the working hand (see "The use of two hands connecting", p. 52).

Sometimes we use the whole body to provide support, particularly for shiatsu in the sitting position.

Mutual support

You will be supported not only by the ground but by the receiver's body. The degree to which you trust in your receiver's physical strength and support will determine the quality of energy they get from you. Support is a two-way process. This leads to a mutual trust that allows relaxation – and this is the moment that leads to change, brought about by the free movement of Ki in your partner's body. The Japanese character for "human being" is like two sticks supporting each other. It conveys the fundamental point that human beings need each other.

Make your partner comfortable on a blanket or carpeted floor. Start from the basic crawling position and move your hands on to the strong parts of your partner's back – the thoracic vertebrae and the sacral region (see below), or the buttocks.

Bring your weight forward slowly until your arms are at right angles to your partner. Lean, applying perpendicular, supporting pressure. Pause for a moment, allowing the stationary aspect of

your pressure to penetrate. Let your own spine relax, and take a breath. Then ease back, move your hands into another comfortable position and lean once more. Your partner will often exhale deeply with your pressure. Don't be afraid – they will breathe in again when they want to.

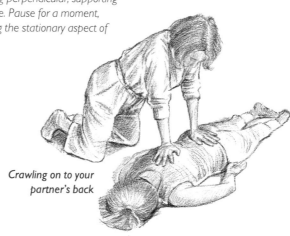

Crawling on to your partner's back

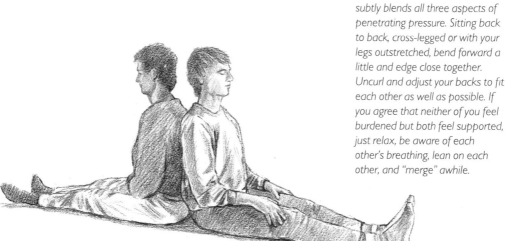

Leaning on your partner

This exercise in mutual support subtly blends all three aspects of penetrating pressure. Sitting back to back, cross-legged or with your legs outstretched, bend forward a little and edge close together. Uncurl and adjust your backs to fit each other as well as possible. If you agree that neither of you feel burdened but both feel supported, just relax, be aware of each other's breathing, lean on each other, and "merge" awhile.

Stretches and rotations

These are an important part of your shiatsu technique. Rotations loosen the joints and position the limbs correctly for working on each Channel. Stretches open up the Channel, activating the Ki; this makes diagnosis easier and treatment more effective.

Stiff and painful joints are the result of blockages in the circulation of Ki and Blood, which do not flow with great ease at the joints, owing to the density of ligaments and tendons that surround the bones. For this reason rotations and stretches are a particularly valuable aspect of treatment.

Once you have practised the exercises below and on page 51 for a while, try to incorporate the principles of advanced shiatsu technique (see pp. 52–5), especially "Keeping your Hara open" and "Visualizing circles".

Arm rotation

Widen your stance for this technique, keeping your nearside knee on the ground and raising the other knee to place your foot on the floor. Grasp firmly round the top of your partner's shoulder with your nearside hand and pick up the wrist with your other, gently shaking the arm to loosen the elbow.

Make a number of circling movements, by carrying the wrist forward, over and above the shoulder, then out to the side and back toward you, gently pulling on your partner's wrist and shoulder to stretch all the joints.

Practise widening the circle toward a full stretch. Move your whole body to follow the action.

Leg rotations

Rotating the leg at the hip, knee, or ankle joints involves many variations of technique depending on which joint is being worked and on the position of the receiver. They are described in detail in the practical routines later in the book. The leg is heavy, so you must always make certain to have a wide base.

Relax your limbs and lift from underneath (see "Relax and keep weight underside" p. 54). Don't strain or pull up from your back.

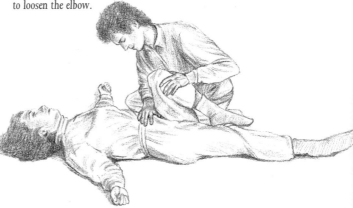

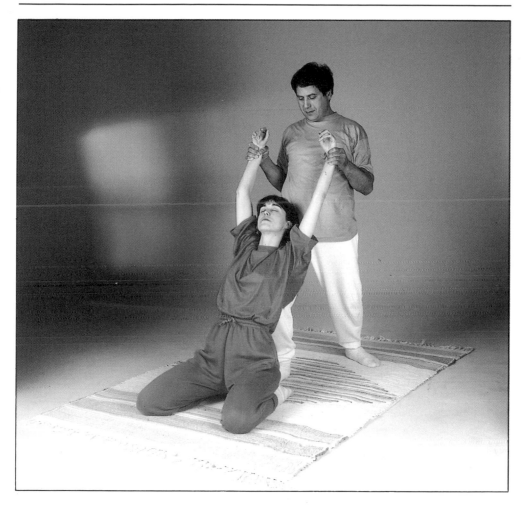

Stretches

These are often incorporated into the rotations, merely by pausing and stretching the limb at a number of points in the circle. Done carefully and without force, they release tension and blockages. They also inform you more fully about the receiver's condition. Lax movements indicate lack of muscle tone or deficient Ki. Tightness or stiffness indicates a local blockage of Ki. Full body stretches (see above) are often used once or twice in a session to release Ki generally and help the receiver to relax.

Full body stretch

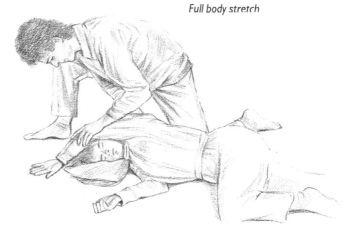

Side position stretch

Principles of advanced technique

From the basic principles and techniques, you can move on to deepen your understanding of the subtle qualities of good shiatsu. This will enhance the experience for the receiver as well as your ability as a practitioner to give good shiatsu. Absorbing these subtle techniques produces great Ki power but can take many years of practice. However, one must start sometime and you are in good company – in Zen there are no experts, only beginners.

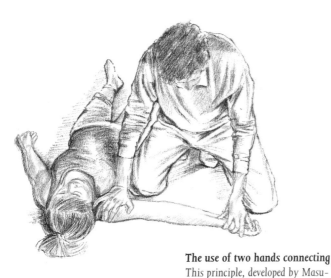

Shiatsu masters say "Two hands feel like one" – the receiver feels something whole and complete. This is good shiatsu.

The use of two hands connecting
This principle, developed by Masunaga, is a unique distingushing feature of Zen shiatsu. Shiatsu encompasses support, a Yin quality; and movement, a Yang, dynamic aspect. Our two hands harmonize the Yin, supportive, and Yang, dynamic, aspects of our work. With practice we begin to feel their unifying power in our partner's response. One hand fulfils the supporting function for both giver and receiver (see "The support hand" on page 49). Remaining stationary, it contacts the receiver's "centres of energy", and is sometimes called the "listening" or "parent" hand. The other, more active hand, sometimes known as the "child", follows the Ki in its movement round the body, innocently exploring the receiver's condition. Either hand can play the supporting roles as required, the important thing being that parent and child are "in touch" with each other (see below).

Continuity
A feeling of flow and continuity is essential to enhance your partner's experience of shiatsu. Continuity depends on your physical movements and the focus of your mind.

Concentrate on the fluent use of your hands as you work around your partner's body. Follow the Ki in its Channels by sliding your active hand along without breaking contact, to feel its condition and locate the tsubos. Move or pause as necessary and always maintain contact with your support hand.

Focus your attention on your partner's breathing, and work from your Hara (see next page).

When your body and mind act in concert, your partner will be unaware of your technique but will experience the shiatsu as being deeply appropriate. Good continuity depends on your ability to work from the Hara.

Working from the Hara

This is the belly or abdomen. It is regarded not only as the physical centre of gravity but as the seat of your constitutional energy or life force, both the origin of Ki and the place where it returns. In Japan, to "have a good Hara" means to be in good health, to have vitality. To be "in Hara" means to be aware of yourself, coordinated and relaxed.

The Hara is nourished by the breath and supported by good diet and digestion, and proper rest.

In practice the Hara is the centre of action. To "move from your Hara" is the epitome of good shiatsu. You can learn to move from your Hara by following "Keeping your Hara open" and "Keeping your weight underside" on page 54. The exercises in Chapter 2 for grounding and breathing will help you to develop Hara consciousness.

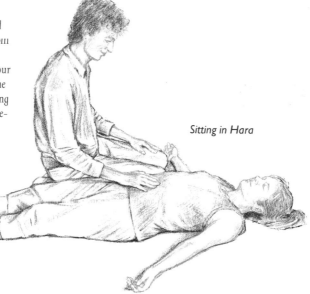

Sitting in Hara

The Tanden and the Mei Mon

The centre of the Hara is a point the width of three fingers below the navel. It is known as the Tanden or "Sea of Ki". A corresponding point, connected to the Tanden via the Kidneys is the Mei Mon, located in the centre of the spine, between the second and third lumbar vertebrae. Also known as "Life Gate" or the "Gate of the Fire of Vitality", the Mei Mon is the seat of Kidney Yang (see p. 80).

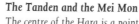

Tanden

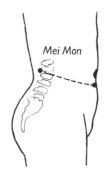

Mei Mon

Relax and keep weight underside

The most important principle of shiatsu is to relax. This does not mean flopping or collapsing, it is merely a reminder to work without effort. Never hunch your back or raise your shoulders and always relax your elbows. Take the easy way and allow your Ki to work for you; it will, if you stay in your Hara. Relaxation connects you with the ground. Keeping weight underside, a principle borrowed from Aikido, is a way of conveying the energy of the ground through your body. Whatever your position, imagine the upper side of your body or limbs are light and the lower aspects heavy — as though being pulled toward Earth. For example: when extending your arm to work with fingers, thumb, or palm, be aware of the heaviness of your elbow. Take energy from the Earth up through your body along all the heavier parts. Lightly direct your Ki with your mind and let the Earth provide both uplift and pulling power. This is the essence of relaxed shiatsu.

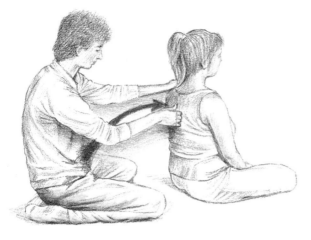

Keeping the weight underside

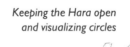

Keeping the Hara open and visualizing circles

Keeping your Hara open

Your aim as a practitioner is to keep your Hara open in all your movements. You can learn to do this by keeping a wide base when giving shiatsu; even in seiza position (see p. 32), have at least the width of a fist between your knees. In this way your actions will flow more easily from the Tanden and you will keep in touch with the receiver's Ki. By keeping your centre of gravity in your Hara, you will also be able to work without losing your balance.

The position of your arms is just as important. If you work too closely you will weaken your Ki power and compensate by using muscular strength, which will tire you.

Visualizing circles

Ki is best conveyed along smooth, open curves. Imagine a flexible sphere in front of your body, encompassed by your arms and chest, and smaller circles supporting your armpits, keeping all the joints open and soft. These will help foster your Ki and at the same time keep your Hara open.

Finding the correct position

By combining all the principles out-lined in this chapter your shiatsu will become an efficient, effective, and enjoyable occupation. All the principles apply at every moment. Practise incorporating them as you work on your partner's body.

Then you will naturally begin to find the right position for you. If you forget the principles you are more likely to make hard work of your shiatsu. There is no absolutely correct posture but the principles are a guide by which you can monitor yourself. The illustrations on this page highlight the difference between working with these principles and trying to work without them.

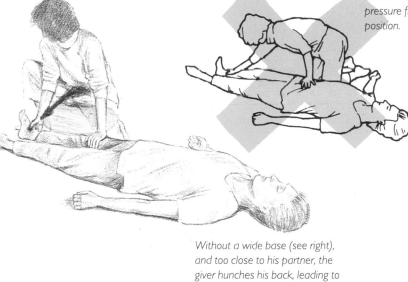

In the illustration below, the giver is over-extending her body, which leads to strain. Her work may feel inconsistent and unsettling. By stepping out to create a wide base (see below, left), the Hara is at her centre of gravity, as it should be. She can lean with perpendicular pressure from a comfortable position.

Without a wide base (see right), and too close to his partner, the giver hunches his back, leading to backache. He cannot thumb correctly because his arm and thumb are bent. He "presses" with his thumb. In the correct position (see left) the giver is balanced and comfortable and works with his thumb and fingers extended. His work will feel more "connected".

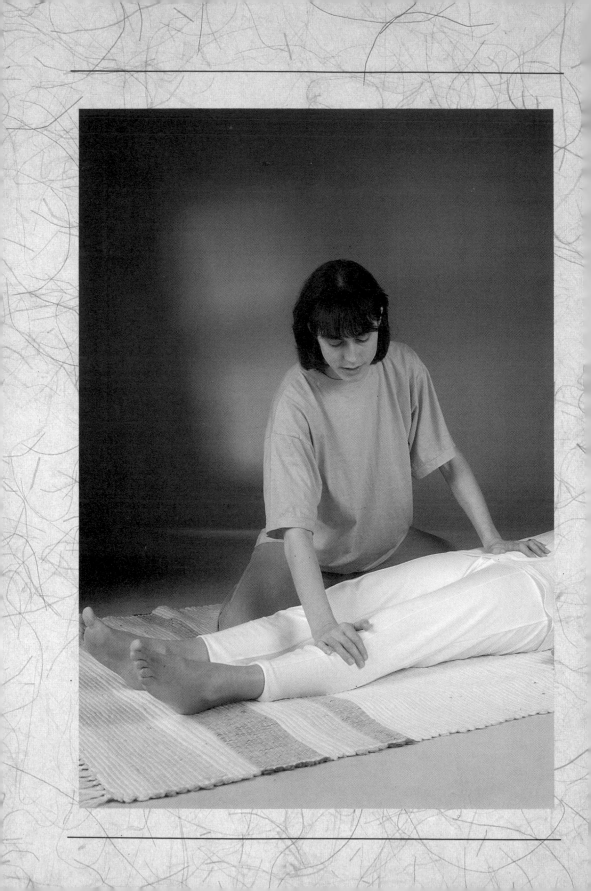

CHAPTER FOUR

The Basic Shiatsu Routine

The active partner is the "giver" of shiatsu from a practical point of view, but communication through physical contact goes both ways. Your hands work and "listen". You will gain physical support from your partner and respond intuitively to his or her feelings, which means that you give and receive at the same time.

Similarly, when you receive shiatsu, you also participate in a two-way process. Allow yourself to feel and respond naturally to any sensations or emotions that arise, and consciously "let go" into the experience. You may feel tense. Sometimes shiatsu can border on the painful, but it should feel like good or helpful pain, never more. Breathe naturally when you feel the pressure and let the tension flow away. Your partner will learn to follow your breathing. Traditionally, learning to receive shiatsu is said to take almost as long as learning to give it.

The best shiatsu sessions are often relaxed, quiet, with few words, but feel free to talk if it seems appropriate. Both the giver and the receiver should give feedback if there is any discomfort or tension. Either partner may have spontaneous insights during a session — share them, they may be valuable; but don't let talking interrupt the continuity.

The basic routine is summarized on pages 58–9. Read the whole chapter before you attempt it. Then, introduce your partner to the space you have prepared for the session and explain what you are going to do. Even if they are already familiar with shiatsu, this ritual will put you both at ease. Ask briefly how your partner is feeling. If you are a bit nervous yourself, why not admit it? A frank exchange of your feelings can ease the situation. Later, your nervousness will disappear. Invite your partner to lie down, then you can begin.

Summary of routine

This basic shiatsu routine, outlined below, covers the whole body. Take care to maintain contact with your partner while changing position: this is comforting and helps to maintain the continuity of your work. Move carefully to avoid bumping your partner.

PRONE POSITION

The routine begins on the upper back. Move from the initial stretch to the lunge position (see p. 61).

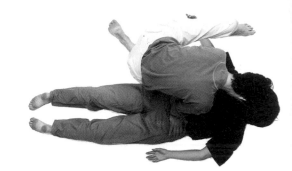

From the back move down to give shiatsu on the nearside leg (see p. 64). Move across your partner to work on the other leg.

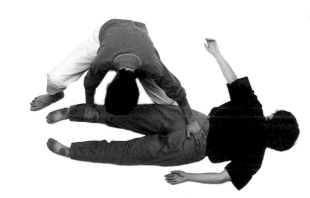

Kneel at your partner's head to finish by working on the shoulders (see pp. 66–7).

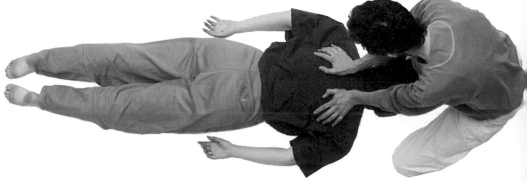

SUPINE POSITION

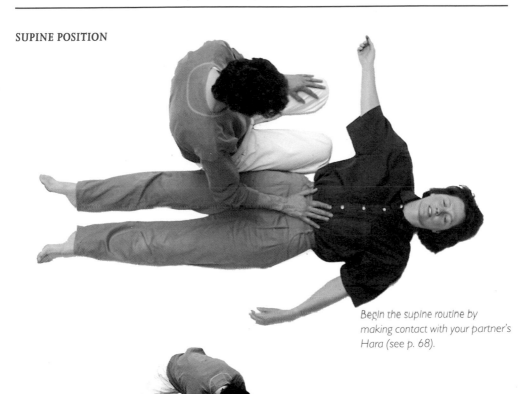

Begin the supine routine by making contact with your partner's Hara (see p. 68).

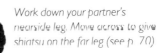

Work down your partner's nearside leg. Move across to give shiatsu on the far leg (see p. 70)

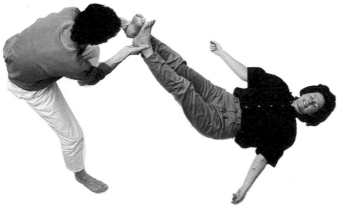

Finish your work on the legs by loosening the hips (see p. 71).

Beginning the basic routine

In the first part of your shiatsu session you will be working with your partner lying face down – the "prone" position. Starting with the back, then the buttocks, the legs, and the feet, you return to the shoulders to finish. Make your partner comfortable, their arms down at their sides so the shoulders rest easily on the floor. A few people will need a pillow in this position (see p. 67) but most will be comfortable with the head turned to one side: remind them to turn it to the other side from time to time to prevent the neck from becoming stiff. Invite them to let you know if you lean or press too hard, as well as to tell you if any place feels particularly good. You can learn a lot from a little feedback.

Working on the back

Most people experience the back and shoulders as a safe part of the body to receive contact. The area is structurally strong, and the Yang Channels, associated with the body's defence, flow downward into it.

Many people suffer from backache, or tension in the shoulders, due to overwork and tiredness. Your partner's back can take your full weight, and, by leaning on it, you will help them "let go" and release tension from tired, aching muscles.

When you are ready, simply rest your hand on any part of your partner's lumbar (lower back) region. Spend a few moments holding your palm gently in place, giving your partner time to adjust to your contact. Start to focus your attention on the depth and rhythm of your partner's breathing.

Stimulating the Ki

Sit in seiza posture next to your partner, if necessary moving their arm a little away from their side to make room for yourself. Breathe into your Hara. Hold your hands at chest level and rub them together briskly and firmly for 30–40 seconds, keeping your shoulders relaxed. This will stimulate the flow of Ki in your whole body, and will warm and sensitize your hands at the start of a session.

Keep your hands joined and your attention focused on how you are feeling for a moment, before making contact with your partner.

Making the first contact

Contact the upper and lower spine
Kneel up, and, with your hand still in contact, turn to face your partner's body. Reposition your hands, one in the sacral region and the other on the back of the chest (thoracic region, see p. 49). Lean forward. Let your spine relax, breathe easily and continue to focus on your partner's breathing for a few moments.

Use the following technique to open the lumbar curve and ease tight muscles before putting direct pressure on the back. Shift your weight back into your hips and knees and bring your upper hand down to the buttock/hip region on the side nearest you. Move your lower hand up to the rib margin on the far side. Lean forward again and use your body weight to create a stretch between your hands. It may help to ask your partner to exhale as you do this.

Hold for a moment, then ease back slightly and bring your hands, one at a time, across to the opposite corresponding positions and repeat the stretch. Do this twice on both sides.

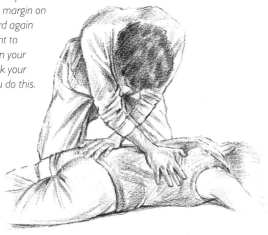

Lumbar cross stretch

Turn to face your partner's head, then place your hands on the upper back, between the shoulder blades, your fingers pointing outward away from each other and the heels of your hands about 1 in (2.5cm) away from each side of the spine (see p. 44). Move your Hara forward, and lean on to your partner's back, using perpendicular pressure. Now ease back and move your hands down, one at a time. Each time they are level, lean forward again to apply perpendicular pressure.

As you approach the lower spine, move your foot out (see below) to work from a wider base. Sink your weight back, with your arms perpendicular to the lower back and sacro-lumbar region. Lean into the position. Now bring your foot closer to finish with

perpendicular pressure on the sacrum. Try to keep these leg movements smooth: your partner will give you the stability you need.

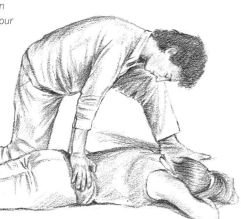

The lunge position

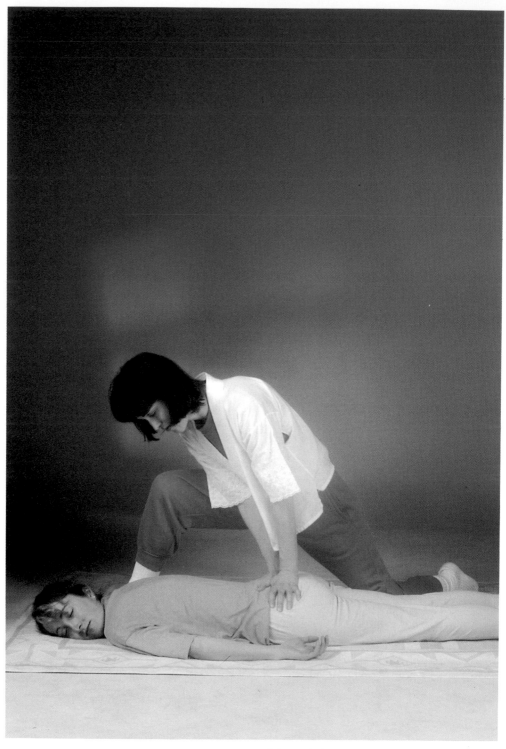

Palming the lower back in the lunge position.

The pelvis and sacro-lumbar region

The area of the buttocks, hips, and pelvis is often affected by stress, poor posture, and a sedentary lifestyle, yet many of us do not recognize the degree to which we accumulate tension here. Tension can produce a misalignment of hips and spine and vice versa.

Basic emotions, such as anger and hatred, affect this area and find expression in kicking and stamping. Our natural sexuality is expressed in pelvic mobility and a natural swinging of the hips. But we restrain all these for much of the time. There are often insufficient healthy avenues for the expression of such natural feelings, but engaging in sports, music, and dancing activities with your friends will help.

Shiatsu can relieve many problems that stem from poor circulation in this area, including backache, sciatica, varicose veins, menstrual pain, bladder troubles, and sexual problems in both men and women.

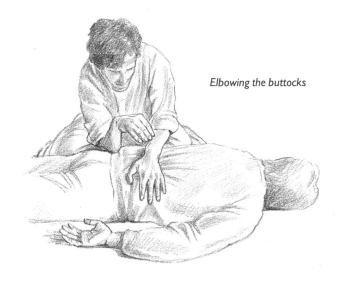

Elbowing the buttocks

The buttock (gluteal) muscles are the largest in the body. They hold a lot of tension, and working them with the thumb is tiring – use elbow technique here. Turn to face your partner and support yourself with one hand on the small of the back (see above). With the flattened elbow of your other arm, lean into the buttock on the near side where you can let your weight sink comfortably, and which allows your partner to relax. Then shift your weight forward into the other buttock, feeling your way into those spots that easily take your weight.

Still leaning gently on your partner for support, step over their thighs. Interlace your fingers and lean into each side of the sacrum, squeezing with the heels of both hands (see right). Reinforce the action by bringing your body forward; you may find it more comfortable to support one elbow with your leg, as shown.

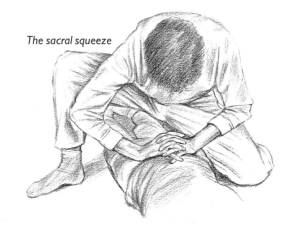

The sacral squeeze

The legs

Improving the energy flow to the legs is an important part of being "grounded". Many people today live almost exclusively "in their heads" – unaware of the tension in their leg muscles, which effectively cuts them off from the ground. High-flying achievers, driven by their intellects, deny themselves the relaxation they need. Dreamers ignore the physical, earth-bound aspects of their reality, and as a result obtain no energy from it, and fail to realize their dreams. Both types may continue in their ways until physical illness demands their attention. Shiatsu can forestall many problems by bringing people back to earth, in touch with their physical body.

Starting the routine

To manage the shiatsu routine on the leg, keep a wide base. Check that your partner's leg is relaxed, the knees and toes turned slightly inward. Place a cushion under the ankles if their legs are stiff.

This is your first chance to practise the principle of "two hands connecting" (see p. 52). Balance and support yourself lightly with one hand on your partner's sacrum and lean forward from your Hara to apply stationary, perpendicular pressure down the leg with the other.

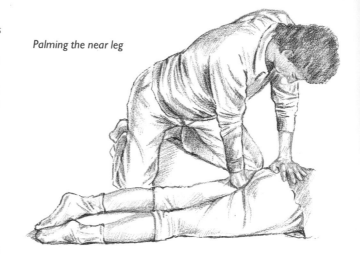

Palming the near leg

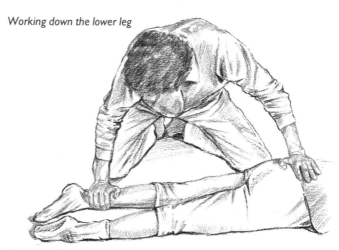

Working down the lower leg

Lean on to the uppermost part of the thigh. Point the fingers outward (see above, top) to avoid the risk of confusing or upsetting your partner by inadvertently touching their genitals. Work down the middle of the leg, directing your pressure straight into the centre. Move your hand down a few inches at a time, easing back toward your haunches whenever you change position.

As you move down the thigh, turn your hand to point the fingers inward. Work gently over the knee. Keeping a wide base, palm down the lower leg to finish above the heel (see above). Apply a medium pressure through the palm or heel of the hand. Keep your hand relaxed to hug the shape of the leg as you proceed (see p. 44).

With your support hand still in place, move over to the far side to palm the other leg in the same way. Swop your support hand as you take up your position on the other side.

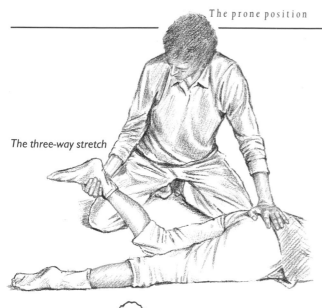

The three-way stretch

The three-way stretch

This stretch works on the hip, knee, and ankle joints to release tension and help the flow of Ki down the leg.

Move back to the first side. With your support hand still resting on the sacrum, reach under your partner's ankle and lift the lower leg (see left), stretching the knee and thigh.

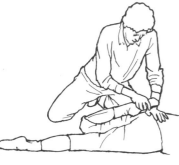

Fold the foot over toward the centre of the buttock (see left). Lean gently but firmly, then slide your hand toward the toes to stretch the foot. Pause for a moment, then carry the foot back out to release the knee joint.

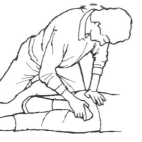

Fold the leg across to the opposite buttock and stretch, following the movement with your body (see left).

The feet

It is important to complete the grounding process by working on your partner's feet. The work you have been doing in the routine so far mainly contacts the Yang Ki, which flows in Channels down the back and outside surfaces from the head. Many shiatsu techniques for the feet help balance Yang with Yin in the whole body.

An easy and most effective technique is to walk or stand on your partner's feet. Try walking forward gradually, up on to the soles, leaning slowly first into one foot then the other (see p. 47). Alternatively, back up on to them with your heels. This will give you a rest from kneeling before you begin the next section.

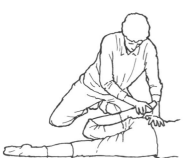

Release the leg and carry it round in a circular movement, bringing the foot toward you and along the nearside of your partner's buttock (see left). Then place the foot on the floor, toes pointing slightly inward. Move to the other side and repeat the 3-way stretch on the other leg.

Natural break

Finishing the routine on the feet provides a natural break for both you and your partner. Both of you will enjoy the pause and you can stretch as you move to the top of your partner's body for the next part of the routine. Before starting work on the back and shoulders, suggest that your partner turn to face the other side. A gentle reminder to do this is worthwhile, because a shiatsu session can be so relaxing that people "forget themselves". It is a shame if a stiff neck detracts from the benefits at the end of your practice.

Upper back and shoulders

We have all experienced tension in the upper back and shoulders. This last part of the prone routine helps to disperse tension and can also benefit the lungs, easing coughs and tightness in the chest. Use the same natural application of your body weight through simple palm and thumb techniques. Relax into them, enjoy yourself, and let the pressure work for both of you.

Making contact with the back

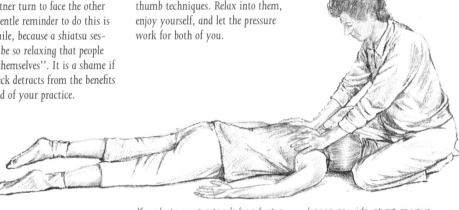

Kneel at your partner's head, at a comfortable distance from them. Too close and your partner will feel oppressed; too far and you will strain, or your pressure will not be perpendicular. Imagine a working circle (see p. 54); kneel with your *knees as wide apart as your partner's ears. Lean comfortably with both hands on the slope of the shoulders. Pause and relax.*

This technique for palming down the back is similar to the one you have already used (see p. 44). Lean into the muscles about 1 in (2.5cm) each side of the spine. Begin near the base of the neck, and palm down between the shoulder blades. Move down the back, one hand at a time, and maintain the perpendicular pressure. Work down to the bottom of the shoulder blades. Pressing here will affect your partner's breathing, but keep your movements smooth and your pressure even.

Palming between the shoulder blades

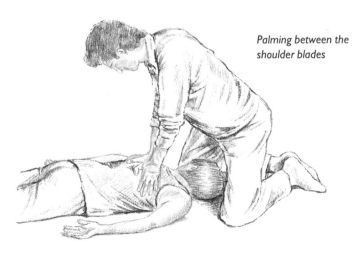

Returning to the top of the back, work with both your thumbs down the muscular ridge about 1 in (2.5cm) each side of the spine. Begin near the most prominent vertebra at the base of the neck and finish level with the base of the shoulder blades.

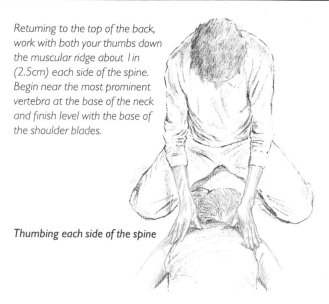

Thumbing each side of the spine

Take a line from the base of the neck along the top of your partner's shoulder. Use the flattened ball of one thumb and work outward in stages to the bony angle at the extremity of the shoulder (see below). Some points may be tender so work carefully. Keep your elbow relaxed and lean in from the hip. Use your other hand for support.

Now take another line about 1 in (2.5cm) lower, giving thumb pressure outward along the muscle between the top of the shoulder and the bony ridge of the shoulder blade. Repeat a few times on each shoulder.

Thumbing across the shoulders

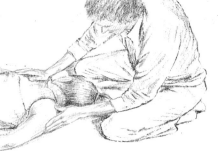

Note

The pressure on the chest and ribs in the prone position may be uncomfortable for some people. Others may have difficulty keeping their neck turned fully to the side. In these cases a pillow under the chest (see right) can provide the solution.

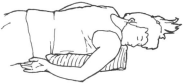

Turning over

To finish your prone routine, rest your hands on your partner's upper back for a moment or two and check how she or he is feeling. Then invite your partner to turn over into the supine position. Stay kneeling where you are during this time. Rest your palms on your partner's forehead or temples for a short while, as a gesture of support and to maintain contact during this transitional phase.

The supine position

Giving shiatsu on the front of the body needs extra consideration. The chest, diaphragm, and belly are centres of emotion and by lying on our backs we are immediately more open, so we may feel exposed and vulnerable. Working face to face can feel intense and involving. Treat your partner with consideration and respect, but continue your shiatsu in an easy, relaxed manner. Good, solid contact can be very strengthening and affirming for your partner. There is no need to be over-cautious.

In this part of the routine, begin by contacting your partner's Hara. Then work on the inner aspect of each arm and hand. Afterwards return to the Hara before giving shiatsu to the legs.

Yin Channels
The Ki of the Yin Organs circulates on the front of the body and on the inner surfaces of the limbs – aspects that are usually protected within the body. The Yin Organs are tradition-ally associated with the emotions in Oriental medicine.

Sit in seiza at your partner's side. Rest your hand on their Hara with your fingertips above, and the heel of the hand below the navel. Relax your arm, do not lean or press. Observe, feel the breathing and just "be" with them for a moment before starting. Even as a beginner, you can contact your partner's Ki at a deep level.

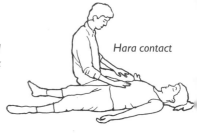

Hara contact

Pick up your partner's arm by the hand or wrist, move your other hand from their Hara to their shoulder and, by leaning back slightly, stretch the arm out. Now move your near hand from the shoulder to the elbow and, carrying the arm, bend and rotate the forearm.

Checking for relaxation
If you feel your partner trying to help you by moving or holding their own arm, gently encourage them to "let go" – something you may often have to repeat when you learn to do the full stretches and rotations. Many people find that giving up control to relax fully with another person is no easy thing.

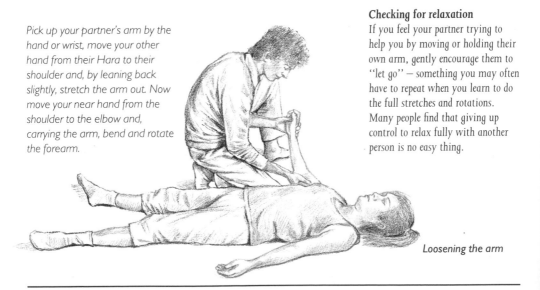

Loosening the arm

Place your partner's arm at a right angle to their side. The palm and inner surface of their arm should be facing up toward you. Then squatting, or kneeling up on your toes, and keeping a wide base, lean with your support hand on to the front of their shoulder. Palm their arm with the other, moving down inch by inch. Keep both hands relaxed, hugging the shape of the limb.

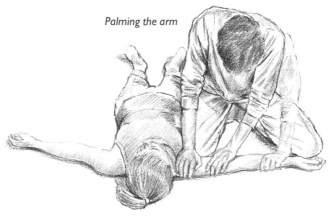

Palming the arm

The Ki is particularly responsive at the hands and feet. Work on the hand is very satisfying and relaxing for the receiver. Give thumb shiatsu to your partner's palm by adopting a special stretching and opening grip: with your partner's fingers toward you, tuck your little fingers through the first space between the fingers, and finger and thumb, on each side of the hand, supporting the back of your partner's hand with your fingers (see near right). Then work with extended thumbs giving pressure systematically over the whole palm (see far right). You can rest the backs of your hands on your knees while you work.

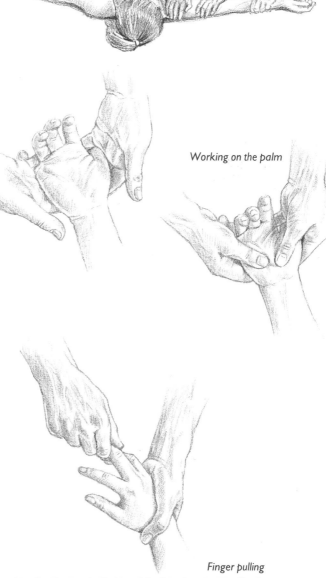

Working on the palm

All the main Channels end or begin on the fingers or toes. The shiatsu technique used to stimulate the Channel endings is to squeeze the sides of the finger firmly between your thumb and the knuckle of your index finger. Work along each finger and thumb in stages from knuckle to fingertip.

Finger pulling

The Ki finds its own direction

Some styles of shiatsu make a rule of following the direction of the Yin and Yang Channels up and down the limbs to "tonify" the Ki. In the Zen style it is considered more important to keep contact with the centre and work outward. The Yin Channels flow up the inner surface of the legs. Yet we always work down the legs, even though this goes "against the flow" of the Ki in the Yin Channels.

The two hands connect and open the Channels and the Ki moves spontaneously if we make good contact and develop "penetrating pressure". We don't need to tell the Ki where to go. It will go there itself!

After working on the arms and hands, return to your partner's Hara. Kneel facing inward as close to your partner's body as possible, knees wide apart. A wide base will help you to work all the way down the leg without over-reaching. Rest one hand comfortably on your partner's Hara and lean the other hand on to the top of the thigh, fingers pointing outward. Kneel up if you need extra height.

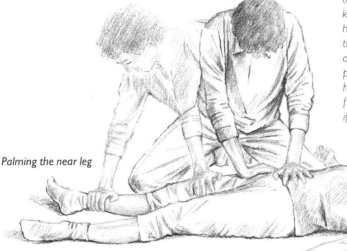

Palming the near leg

Palm the near side of the leg past the knee to the ankle, moving in stages, sliding the hand along between points to keep contact. On the lower leg, give more pressure to the outside of the shinbone through the heel of the hand, fingertips curled naturally over for support.

Bring your weight forward to palm down the inner aspect of the far leg. Keep the pressure of your support hand constant on the Hara as you rock back and forward to move and give pressure with your active hand. Palm down from thigh to ankle. Then move round to repeat the work on the other aspects of the legs from the other side.

The feet

After palming the legs, move down to the feet. You can finish by simply grasping both feet below the ankle and squeezing all the way down the sides, leaning back and stretching them down a little as you do so. Or you can attempt, with care, and your mind on your Hara, the stretching and loosening sequence for the waist and lower spine.

Palming the far leg

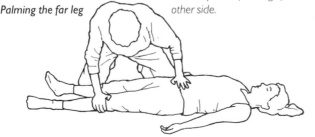

Squat down close to your partner's feet, your knees wide outside your arms and your back as straight as possible. Reach down behind your partner's ankles to lift their heels a fraction off the floor (see below). Pause and breathe.

Raising the feet

In one smooth movement, keeping your back as straight as possible, exhale as you straighten your knees to lift your partner's legs about 30 degrees and step in a little to rest your arms on your thighs (see below). Anchored by your partner's body weight, lean back to stretch the spine, while you relax and breathe.

Resting on your thighs

Swinging the legs

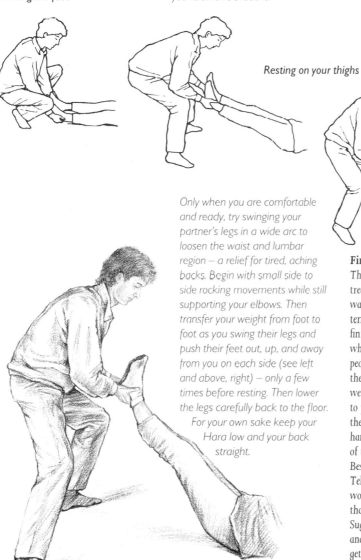

Only when you are comfortable and ready, try swinging your partner's legs in a wide arc to loosen the waist and lumbar region – a relief for tired, aching backs. Begin with small side to side rocking movements while still supporting your elbows. Then transfer your weight from foot to foot as you swing their legs and push their feet out, up, and away from you on each side (see left and above, right) – only a few times before resting. Then lower the legs carefully back to the floor. For your own sake keep your Hara low and your back straight.

Finishing the routine

The way you finish your shiatsu treatments is as important as the way you begin. There is no set pattern for shiatsu routines. Often we finish on the feet, as in this routine, which is very good for grounding people. But sometimes the hands or the head and neck are the last areas we work. Then, as well as speaking to your partner, use touch to signal the end. A short pause followed by a hand on their shoulder or a squeeze of their wrist conveys the message. Best of all is to contact the Hara. Tell your partner gently that the work is done for now. You may find that they have become very relaxed. Suggest that they open their eyes and re-orient themselves before slowly getting up. Ask them how they feel. Give them time!

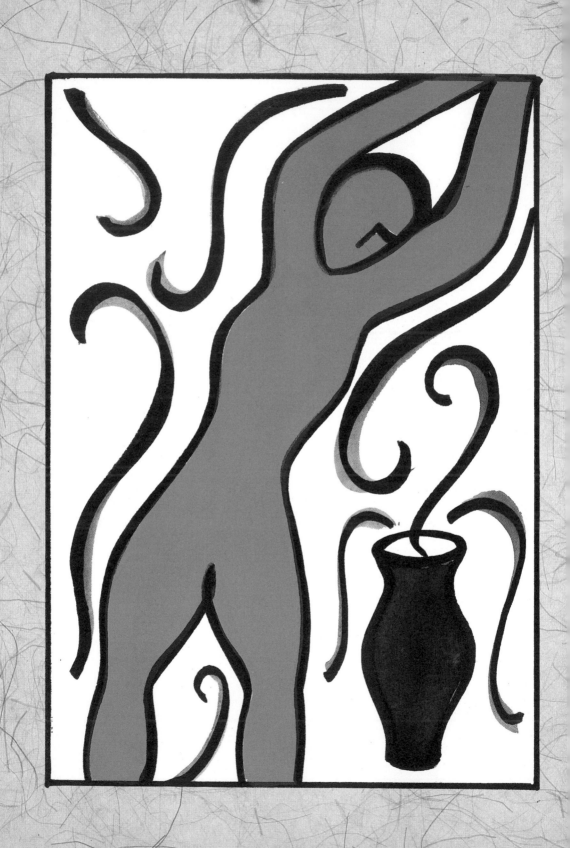

PART TWO

Pathways of Ki

WORKING ON THE CHANNELS

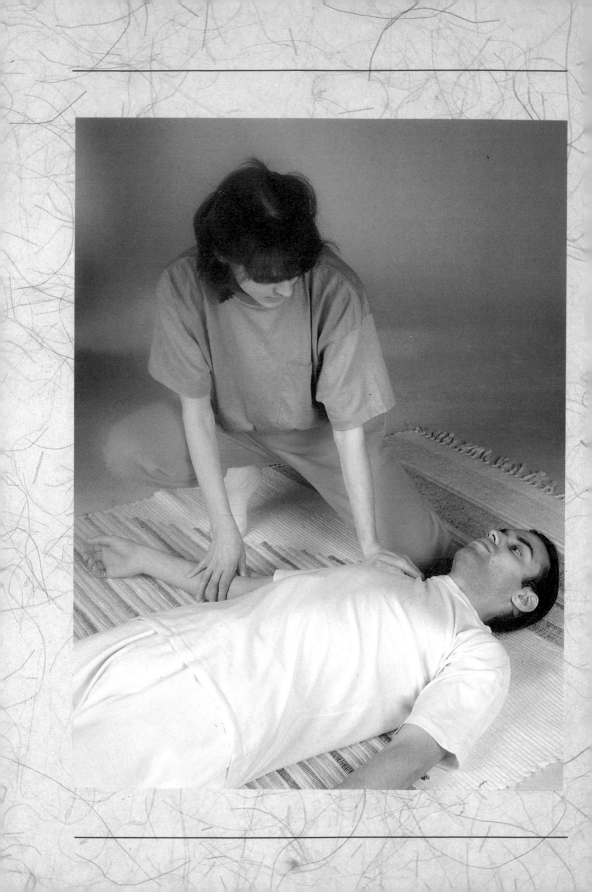

CHAPTER FIVE

Patterns of Ki

From ancient times the Chinese interpreted the behaviour of Ki from its manifestations. Areas of pain, swelling, irritation, or redness that arose in illness were seen as disturbances or blockages of Ki on the body surface. It was found that some conditions, even internal ones, could be ameliorated by pressing or rubbing these tender areas. Other "points of pain" were discovered in the process that also seemed to bring benefit when pressed. The use of points was fairly random at first, but certain of them were repeatedly found helpful for similar conditions and, as more were added, they were recorded and systemized. Through experience it became clear that all aspects of the body were interrelated, and the theory arose that the points were linked by a network of subtle interconnecting Channels. These conducted Ki to all parts inside the body and to the skin on the outside. Twelve primary Channels came to be associated with the body's main Organs.

Symptoms and signs of disease can be seen as part of a pattern, manifesting disharmony of Ki in particular Channels. They reflect either a dysfunction of a corresponding Organ or a disturbance of the body along the course of the Channels.

The major Channels flow near to the surface and can be influenced through shiatsu at points along their path, reharmonizing the Organs and restoring and maintaining balance in the whole system. The study of the Channels is an essential step in transforming your shiatsu from a general treatment, which may be relaxing or stimulating, into a more precise and effective means of healing.

The major Channels are illustrated on pages 76–7, and the nature of the points, or "tsubos", is described on page 78. The sequence of the Channels, and the cyclical movement of their Ki are explained on page 79. Pages 80–1 summarize the functions of the Organs.

The major Channels

Ki is distributed throughout the body by an intricate web of subtle Channels. Twelve "primary Channels" connect the Organs and flow near the surface in pathways on the sides of the head and trunk and along the limbs. Most of the classical acupuncture points are found along the primary Channels.

Eight "extra Channels" circulate a little deeper, intersecting with the twelve primary Channels, and acting as reservoirs of Ki. A network of subsidiary Channels completes the system.

Two of the extra Channels, the "mid line" Channels, have their own points and may be included with the primary Channels. Together, these fourteen "major Channels" are the subjects of this book.

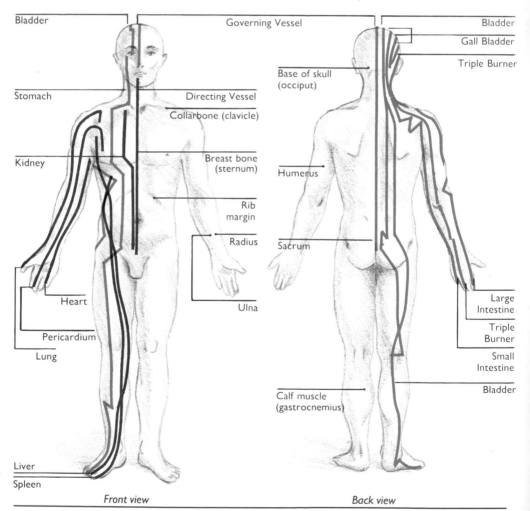

Bladder

Stomach

Kidney

Heart

Pericardium

Lung

Liver

Spleen

Front view

Governing Vessel

Directing Vessel

Collarbone (clavicle)

Breast bone (sternum)

Rib margin

Radius

Ulna

Base of skull (occiput)

Humerus

Sacrum

Calf muscle (gastrocnemius)

Bladder

Gall Bladder

Triple Burner

Large Intestine

Triple Burner

Small Intestine

Bladder

Back view

The mid line Channels

Thumb and finger pressure can be given to points along the mid line Channels, but it is usual to keep in touch with these Channels during a shiatsu session with the support hand (see p. 49). Maintain contact in this way on the Hara, chest, or lower back, while the active hand works outward from these areas. By keeping the support hand on the mid line Channels, the central circulation of Ki is connected to the primary Channels.

The mid line Channels, also known as the "Governing Vessel" and the "Directing Vessel", control all the others. The Governing Vessel runs up the spine and over the head. It controls all the Yang Channels. The Yin Channels are regulated by the Directing Vessel, which follows the mid line over the abdomen and chest up to the throat and mouth.

Key to Channel abbreviations used in the book

Lu	Lung
LI	Large Intestine
St	Stomach
Sp	Spleen
H	Heart
SI	Small Intestine
Bl	Bladder
K	Kidney
P	Pericardium
TB	Triple Burner
GB	Gall Bladder
Liv	Liver
DV	Directing Vessel
GV	Governing Vessel

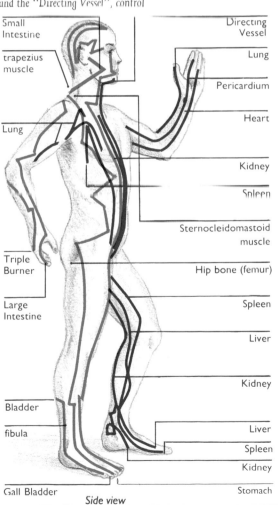

Small Intestine
trapezius muscle
Lung
Triple Burner
Large Intestine
Bladder
fibula
Gall Bladder

Directing Vessel
Lung
Pericardium
Heart
Kidney
Spleen
Sternocleidomastoid muscle
Hip bone (femur)
Spleen
Liver
Kidney
Liver
Spleen
Kidney
Stomach

Side view

The superficial pathways of all the major Channels are shown most clearly in the front, back, and side views. The Yin Channels, shown in blue, flow from the feet up to the chest and out to the fingertips. The Yang Channels, shown in orange, are, with the exception of the Stomach Channel (see p. 88), all located on the back and outer surfaces of the limbs. They flow from the hands to the head and downward to the feet.

Naming the Channels

The full name for each Channel is derived from the Organ to which it is connected, the limb along which it runs, the time of its activity, its position on the arm or leg, and its polarity (Yin or Yang).

So, for example, the full name for the Lung Channel is **Lung Channel, arm Greater Yin.**

Classical points

Nearly all of the 365 classical points or "tsubos", situated along the 14 Channels, were established by the time of The Yellow Emperor's Classic of Internal Medicine — the earliest Chinese medical work. Over centuries of experience these became recognized for their predictable influence over certain functions and parts of the body.

Chinese characters

Chinese characters are a visual representation of objects or ideas. You can see from the illustrations (below) how the characters for pressure point, or "tsubo", and "Channel" describe the parts of their structure.

A tsubo

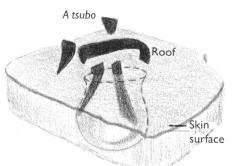

A tsubo is a pressure point, where the Ki can gather — a "hollow" or "opening" where the Ki can be reached and influenced by applying pressure. Its structure is more three-dimensional than the word "point" suggests.

Some points reacted to certain diseases, becoming irritated, and tender when pressed. Because of this, they could be used for diagnosis as well as treatment. Groups of points with similar characteristics were subsequently linked, and the system of Channels became established.

However, the older system of treating any points of pain or tenderness remained in the tradition. The Chinese call these points "Ah Shi" points, meaning "that's it!", as a response to touching the affected part. Shiatsu treatment is not confined to classical acupuncture points: look for the "hollows" or points of deepest penetration that feel satisfying to the receiver. This is where you can work on the Ki.

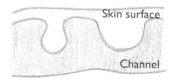

Normal tsubos

Tsubos are like openings into the Channel. Your pressure is accepted. Ki responds. Your partner feels comforted and supported. Even pain is pleasant pain. Some tsubos are more lax, or open, than others.

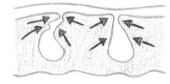

Blocked tsubos

Physical tension blocks Ki and produces distorted or closed tsubos that are difficult to penetrate (see pp. 162–3). Pressure on these points can be uncomfortable or painful. Do not work here for long; you will tire, and your partner will not benefit.

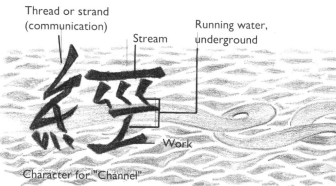

Character for "Channel"

The Chinese were fond of using water as a metaphor for Ki. The Channels are like water courses and the points are like eddies, vortices, or swirls in the current. Both Channels and points are found in the spaces between the muscles and other tissues of the body. These tissues are like the banks of a river: it is the water that creates the Channel, but the banks influence the flow.

The "Chinese Clock"

According to tradition, Ki flows through the 12 primary Channels in a given order. The Chinese Clock (see right) represents the path of Ki as it passes through the Channels. Its passage takes the Ki through Yin and Yang Organs in pairs: the Lung Channel (Yin) is paired with the Large Intestine Channel (Yang), and so on. Each Yin and Yang pair of Organs belongs to the same Element (see below and p. 25).

The activity of Ki intensifies in each Channel successively in a wave-like movement through the system, completing a cycle every 24 hours. Therefore each Channel has a peak of activity lasting 2 hours and a correspondingly low phase 12 hours later. This is significant as observing the time of day when symptoms appear may indicate a disharmony of the relevant Channel. The model also highlights favoured times for certain exercises or activities in maintaining health.

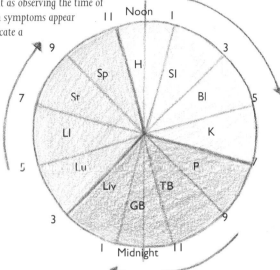

Diagrammatic representation of the cycle of Ki

This diagram represents the movement of Ki through successive pairs of Yin and Yang Channels. It flows in a cycle that begins with the Lung Channel, emerging on the outer chest, then follows a continuous sequence. The sequence finishes with the Liver Channel, where the Ki rejoins the Lung Channel for the cycle to begin again. Each Yin Channel connects with its Yang counterpart on the hand or the foot. All the Yin Channels meet on the chest, the Yang Channels meet on the head.

The Yin and Yang Channels can be divided into three groups of four, each group having a Yin–Yang pair on the arm, and another Yin–Yang pair on the leg. Each Yin–Yang pair belongs to the same element. The routines demonstrated in Chapters 6, 7, and 8, work on the Channels in their groups of four.

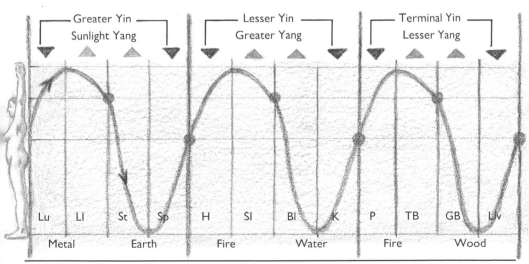

The Yin and Yang Organs and their Channels

Traditional Oriental physiology and anatomy record a very different view of the body from that of modern Western medicine. The Yin and Yang Organs that form the core of the system are described in terms of their functions and interrelationships rather than their physical location, shape, structure, or chemistry. A significant example is the Triple Burner, an Organ in Chinese medicine, which has specific functions, harmonizing the upper, middle, and lower parts of the body, but has no physical counterpart (see also p. 132). Chinese medicine ascribes a much wider role to each of the Organs than does modern physiology, and their related Channels integrate the parts with the whole. Observation of patterns and connections, rather than analysis of component parts, has always been the way of Oriental medicine. Understanding their fundamental characteristics will help you recognize more easily which Organs are implicated in any illness, and the nature of the particular underlying imbalance.

Functions of the Yin Organs

There are five Yin Organs — the Lungs, Spleen, Heart, Kidneys, and Liver. Known as the "solid" Organs, they share the Yin characteristics of being internal, deep, and hidden. Yin Organs are the most important in the body; they are responsible for the transformation, circulation, and storage of Ki and Blood — pure substances essential to the body. Each of these Organs has Yin or Yang characteristics in varying degrees. Their functions are expressed in the quality and direction of movement of their Ki. Some are more concerned with Ki, some with Blood; some are situated higher in the body, some lower. The Lungs are on top, like a lid, and act downward. The Kidneys are at the bottom, and like roots, they hold and store Ki, but also send it upward. The Spleen also sends Ki up, while the Liver smooths and eases the flow of Ki whatever its direction.

Functions of the Yang Organs

The Yang Organs assist the Yin. Yang relates more to the surface or outside of things and generally the Yang or "hollow" Organs are those that make up the digestive tract. Defined only by their outer walls, they are concerned with receiving and processing food and eliminating waste. In this sense they connect with the outside and their contents are unrefined — not yet usable by the body, or surplus to its needs. The Gall Bladder is the exception; it is a hollow Organ that stores a pure body fluid, bile, which helps digestion.

The Lungs receive the air, transform the Ki of air and food into Human Ki. They disperse Ki to the skin for defence, circulate Ki in the Channels and send surplus Ki down to be stored by the Kidneys.

The Liver stores Blood and eases all movements of Ki.

The Gall Bladder stores bile and assists the liver.

The Stomach receives food and drink. It sends the purest parts to the Spleen and the less pure down to the Small Intestine. Stomach Ki goes down.

The Small Intestine separates and absorbs pure fluids and passes on impure fluids to the Bladder and impure solids to the Large Intestine.

The Bladder stores and excretes the waste fluids.

The Large Intestine excretes the solid waste after absorbing fluids.

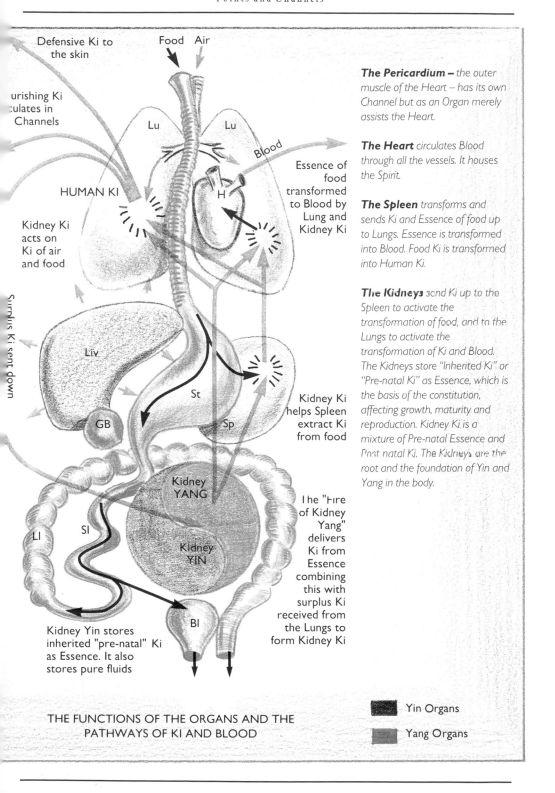

Defensive Ki to the skin

Food   Air

urishing Ki
culates in
Channels

Lu   Lu

Blood

HUMAN KI

Kidney Ki
acts on
Ki of air
and food

Surplus Ki sent down

Liv

St

GB

Sp

H

Essence of
food
transformed
to Blood by
Lung and
Kidney Ki

Kidney Ki
helps Spleen
extract Ki
from food

Kidney
YANG

Kidney
YIN

LI   SI

Bl

Kidney Yin stores
inherited "pre-natal" Ki
as Essence. It also
stores pure fluids

The "Fire
of Kidney
Yang"
delivers
Ki from
Essence
combining
this with
surplus Ki
received from
the Lungs to
form Kidney Ki

The Pericardium – the outer muscle of the Heart – has its own Channel but as an Organ merely assists the Heart.

The Heart circulates Blood through all the vessels. It houses the Spirit.

The Spleen transforms and sends Ki and Essence of food up to Lungs. Essence is transformed into Blood. Food Ki is transformed into Human Ki.

The Kidneys send Ki up to the Spleen to activate the transformation of food, and to the Lungs to activate the transformation of Ki and Blood. The Kidneys store "Inherited Ki" or "Pre-natal Ki" as Essence, which is the basis of the constitution, affecting growth, maturity and reproduction. Kidney Ki is a mixture of Pre-natal Essence and Post natal Ki. The Kidneys are the root and the foundation of Yin and Yang in the body.

THE FUNCTIONS OF THE ORGANS AND THE
PATHWAYS OF KI AND BLOOD

Yin Organs

Yang Organs

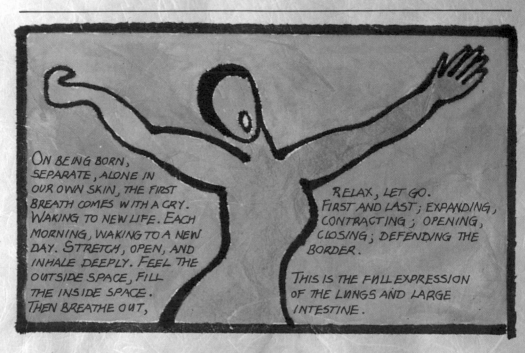

ON BEING BORN,
SEPARATE, ALONE IN
OUR OWN SKIN, THE FIRST
BREATH COMES WITH A CRY.
WAKING TO NEW LIFE. EACH
MORNING, WAKING TO A NEW
DAY. STRETCH, OPEN, AND
INHALE DEEPLY. FEEL THE
OUTSIDE SPACE, FILL
THE INSIDE SPACE.
THEN BREATHE OUT,

RELAX, LET GO.
FIRST AND LAST; EXPANDING,
CONTRACTING; OPENING,
CLOSING; DEFENDING THE
BORDER.

THIS IS THE FULL EXPRESSION
OF THE LUNGS AND LARGE
INTESTINE.

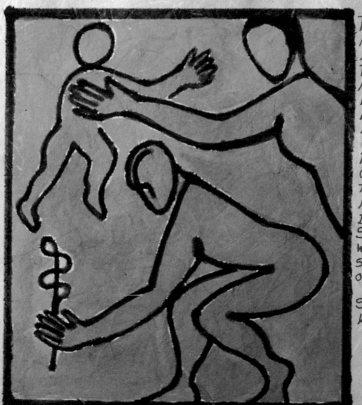

THE CHILD REACHES TO ITS
MOTHER FOR SUSTENANCE
AND WARMTH.
THE MOTHER REACHES
FORWARD TO HOLD AND
ENFOLD THE CHILD.
LATER WE MUST LOOK
FURTHER AFIELD FOR
OUR NEEDS.
BECOME A HUNTER-
GATHERER, SENSES
TUNED; SEEK SPECIAL
INFORMATION, LEARN
DISCRIMINATION.
SHOPPING, OR PICKING
WILD FRUITS AND HERBS;
STUDYING, OR REACHING
OUT FOR CONTACT.

STOMACH AND SPLEEN
KI - ALWAYS IN FRONT.

CHAPTER SIX

The Front Channels

LUNGS · LARGE INTESTINE
STOMACH · SPLEEN

This chapter, and the two that follow, each look at two pairs of Organs that are linked to each other in their work. They describe the functions of the pathways of their Channels (see pp. 84-5 and 88-9), illustrate exercises for each pair of Organs (see pp. 86-7 and 90 1), and end with a detailed routine for working on each group of Channels (see pp. 92-103).

The four Channels in this chapter are the first four in the cycle of Ki (see p. 79). As a group, they deal with our need to absorb energy and sustenance from the environment after birth, and to discharge and return what is not required. Each of the Channels can be worked with your partner lying face up - the supine position.

The images on the facing page evoke archetypal bodily expressions of the quality of Ki in each pair of Organs. In this chapter, the Lungs and Large Intestine are the first pair of Organs (see top, facing page). They open to the outside and control the border between inside and out. The Lungs take energy in from the air and expel waste gases. They also control the skin, which "breathes". The Large Intestine absorbs fluid and excretes solid wastes.

The second pair of Organs, the Stomach and Spleen, are the Organs of digestion (see bottom, facing page). Their Channels flow over the front of the body. The Spleen opens to the mouth and controls taste. The Stomach Channel passes through the centre of the breast. To the suckling infant, mouth, nipple, and warm embrace are all one thing. So begins our association of food and drink with security and comfort.

Once you have learned the pathways and points (tsubos) in this chapter and the two that follow, you will have the basics from which to build your own routines. Remember to work with the principles and techniques described earlier in this book.

The Lung Channel pathway

The Lung Channel begins deep in the solar plexus region (the Middle Burner, see p. 132) and descends to meet the Large Intestine, the Yang Organ paired with the Lungs. Winding up past the Stomach, it crosses the diaphragm, divides, and enters the Lungs. It then re-unites, passes up the middle of the windpipe to the throat and divides again, surfacing in the hollow region near the front of the shoulder (Lu 1). From here it passes over the shoulder and down the anterior (front) aspect of the arm along the outer border of the biceps muscle. It reaches the outside of the biceps tendon in the elbow crease (Lu 5), and continues down the forearm to the wrist just above the base of the thumb (Lu 9). The Channel crosses the height of the thumb muscle to finish at the corner of the thumbnail.

THE LUNG CHANNEL
Arm Greater Yin

Internal pathway symptoms
Throat problems, loss of voice, asthma, breathlessness, bronchitis, bowel problems - constipation, colitis, etc

Lu 1
"Central Residence"
Helps Lung Ki descend.
Acute cough, asthma, and tight chest

Lu 5
"Foot Marsh"
Cools and calms. *For harsh, dry cough*

Lu 9
"Greater Abyss"
Strengthens Lungs.
For weakness and chronic Lung troubles

Lu 10
"Fish Border"
Painful, sore throat

The Lung Channel — functions and associated symptoms

The Lungs rule Ki. They receive, transform, and distribute it in the body; to the skin for defence, through the Channels to nourish and energize all parts, and down to all the other Organs, especially the Kidneys, where surplus post-natal Ki adds to our constitutional reserves.

If the Lungs are weak they cannot supply enough Ki to the skin for defence; climatic influences can then invade through the pores. This according to Oriental medicine is how we "catch" chills, colds, fevers,

and stiff neck from sitting in a draught. A chronic weakness of the Lungs generally produces tiredness, often breathlessness, and a pale complexion. If the Lungs cannot circulate Ki, it accumulates, producing a tight, stuffy chest and a cough, or asthma.

Other Lung symptoms may need treatment on more than one Channel; for example, a dry, irritating cough, dry throat, and dry skin often require work on the Kidney Channel as well.

Channel symptoms

Pain and other symptoms occurring along the superficial course of a Channel are called "Channel symptoms". They will benefit from work on the Channel. In the Lung Channel these include chest and shoulder pains, pain along the arm or in the thumb, and stiff neck.

THE LARGE INTESTINE CHANNEL
Arm Sunlight Yang

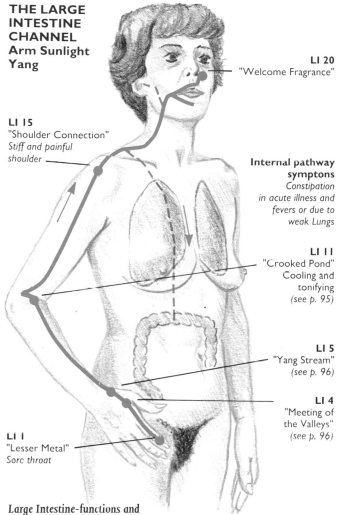

LI 20
"Welcome Fragrance"

LI 15
"Shoulder Connection"
Stiff and painful shoulder

Internal pathway symptons
Constipation in acute illness and fevers or due to weak Lungs

LI 11
"Crooked Pond"
Cooling and tonifying
(see p. 95)

LI 5
"Yang Stream"
(see p. 96)

LI 4
"Meeting of the Valleys"
(see p. 96)

LI 1
"Lesser Metal"
Sore throat

The Large Intestine Channel pathway

The Large Intestine Channel begins by the outside corner of the index fingernail. It runs along the edge of the finger, between the two tendons of the thumb at the wrist joint (LI 5) and along the bony margin of the outer edge of the arm (the radius bone) to the elbow. The point LI 11 is situated at the outside of the elbow crease, which is visible when the arm is bent. From here the Channel continues to the point LI 15 on the outside of the shoulder muscle. It then crosses the shoulder blade and meets the Governing Vessel below the 7th cervical vertebra at point GV 14. It descends internally to connect first with the Lung and then with its own Organ, the Large Intestine. From the shoulder a branch travels upward over the muscle at the side of the neck (sterno-cleido-mastoid) to the cheek, passing through the lower gums, then round over the top lip. It terminates beside the opposite nostril, where it links to the Stomach Channel.

Large Intestine-functions and associated symptoms

The Large Intestine receives the remaining part of food and drink from the Small Intestine, absorbs more fluids, and excretes the residue. It can be unbalanced by improper diet, acute illness, weakness, or worry, although these are often better treated indirectly through a related Channel, rather than by the Large Intestine Channel itself.

For example, many bowel troubles will respond better to treatment of the Lung, Kidney, Spleen, or Stomach Channels. For problems created by worry, or constipation associated with weakness or breathlessness, treat the Lungs. Weak or chilly people are often prone to watery stools or diarrhoea, with rumblings, distension, and abdominal discomfort. In this case treat the Spleen, which controls transformation of fluids.

Treat the Large Intestine Channel for shoulder pain and tennis elbow, and blockages or pain in the sensory organs, including nasal congestion, sinusitis, or toothache. Work on this Channel from elbow to hand for constipation that is due to heat or fever.

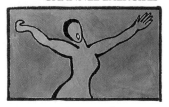

CHANNEL EXERCISES

Lungs and Large Intestine

The Oriental tradition of doing exercises for longevity and health includes some that strengthen particular Organs and improve the flow of Ki in the Channels. A few such exercises are given below for the Lungs and Large Intestine.

A common thread in all traditional exercises is the importance attached to the breath. Good breathing is the source of our vitality. The Lungs govern respiration, rule Ki, and open into the nose. The Large Intestine Channel finishes at the nose and helps regulate breathing. Nowadays people suffer greatly from obstructed nasal passages, allergic sinusitis, and general problems from polluted city air and air "conditioning".

Refined, processed, and de-natured foods weaken the Large Intestine and are often linked with allergies, and both Lung and Large Intestine are affected by worry and stress, and the effects of sedentary living. Walking, swimming, cycling, and hill climbing, as well as formal exercises and deep nasal breathing, counter many of these negative influences.

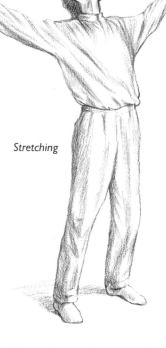

Stretching

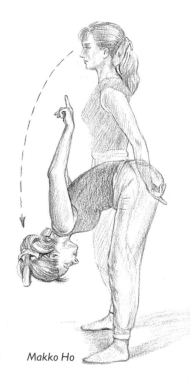

Makko Ho stretches
Masunaga adopted a series of stretches for each pair of Channels from the Japanese exercise system known as Makko Ho. These have become widely associated with shiatsu — good for givers and receivers alike.

Yawning boosts the oxygen in the Blood. To induce a yawn, rub your face next to your mouth and nose, then stretch and open your mouth. Breathe in as you raise your arms, then circle them round, looking upward. Pause for a moment with your arms stretched back (see above). Feel the Ki flow along the Channels. Exhale as you lower your arms.

For the Lungs and Large Intestine, stand with feet apart. Link your thumbs behind you, then exhale and bend forward from your hips, stretching your arms out and up, knees slightly bent (see right). Breathe and relax further into it for a few breaths. Uncurl slowly as you exhale.

Makko Ho

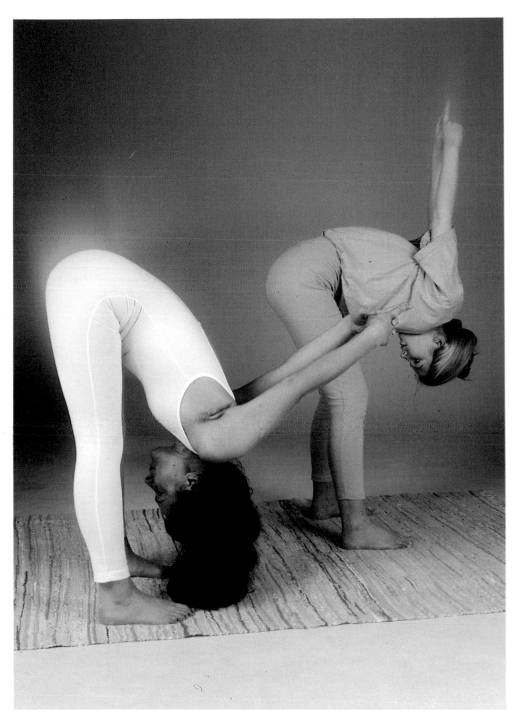

Stretching the Lung and Large Intestine Channels – the Makko Ho Stretch

The Stomach Channel pathway

Starting beside the nose, near LI 20, the Stomach Channel meets the Bladder Channel at point Bl 1 on the forehead. From St 1, just below the eye, it passes into the upper gums and round the mouth to link with the Governing and Directing Vessels. Next, via the lower gums, it ascends in front of the ear to the forehead.

From the jaw it descends alongside the throat to the collarbone region, where an internal branch descends to meet the Stomach and Spleen. The superficial path continues down over the abdomen to the pubic area, where a second internal branch from the Stomach rejoins it.

The Channel continues down the anterior thigh, passing just to the outside of the kneecap. At St 36, below the knee, the Channel divides again. The surface branch runs down the leg beside the shinbone, ending on the outside of the second toe. The deeper branch descends to the middle toe. From the top of the foot a connection runs to the Spleen Channel.

The Stomach and Spleen in digestion

The Stomach and the Spleen share the role of digestion and are often considered and treated together. Ki from food is the basis of the body's Ki and Blood, so it is important to strengthen both Stomach and Spleen in any chronic illness.

The Stomach suffers most from dryness and heat. It "likes wetness and dislikes dryness". If its fluids are deficient, digestion will suffer and the mouth and lips will become dry. The Stomach directs Ki downward. If disturbed the Ki may "rebel" upward causing nausea, vomiting, or headaches.

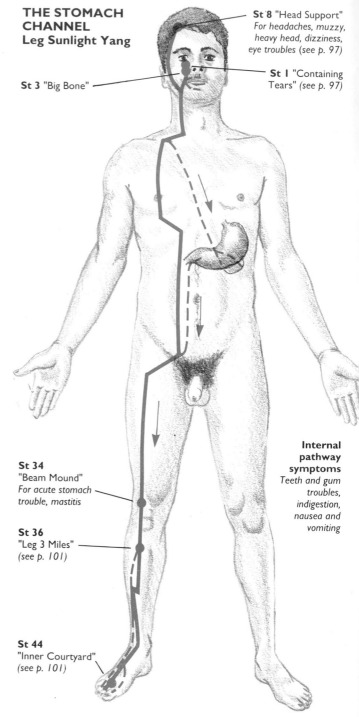

THE STOMACH CHANNEL
Leg Sunlight Yang

St 3 "Big Bone"

St 8 "Head Support"
For headaches, muzzy, heavy head, dizziness, eye troubles (see p. 97)

St 1 "Containing Tears" (see p. 97)

St 34
"Beam Mound"
For acute stomach trouble, mastitis

St 36
"Leg 3 Miles"
(see p. 101)

St 44
"Inner Courtyard"
(see p. 101)

Internal pathway symptoms
Teeth and gum troubles, indigestion, nausea and vomiting

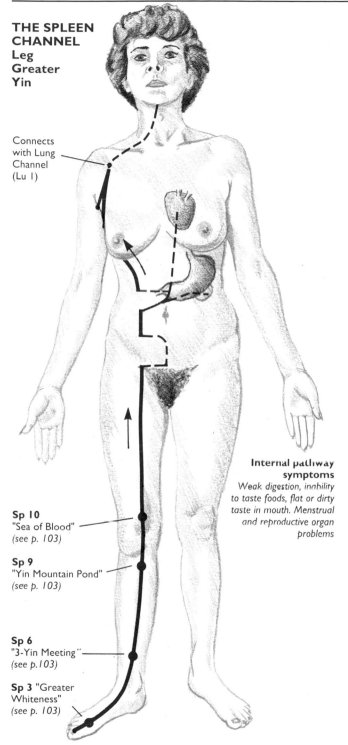

**THE SPLEEN
CHANNEL
Leg
Greater
Yin**

Connects
with Lung
Channel
(Lu 1)

**Internal pathway
symptoms**
*Weak digestion, inability
to taste foods, flat or dirty
taste in mouth. Menstrual
and reproductive organ
problems*

Sp 10
"Sea of Blood"
(see p. 103)

Sp 9
"Yin Mountain Pond"
(see p. 103)

Sp 6
"3-Yin Meeting"
(see p.103)

Sp 3 "Greater
Whiteness"
(see p. 103)

The Spleen Channel pathway

*Beginning on the inside tip of the big
toe, the Spleen Channel follows the
inner aspect of the foot to the arch,
then turns up in front of the inner
ankle to Sp 6. It continues up the
leg, just behind the bone, crossing
the knee and ascending the anterior
thigh from the inner border of the
kneecap.*

*From the groin it enters the
lower abdomen, meets the Directing
Vessel, then resurfaces briefly before
penetrating the Spleen and Stomach.
The main Channel then ascends
through the diaphragm, over the
chest, and crosses the Lung Channel
at Lu 1. It continues up to the
oesophagus and under the tongue. An
inner branch from the Stomach region transports Ki up to the Heart.*

The functions of the Spleen

The principal role of the Spleen is
transforming and transporting. It
transforms food and conveys the
nourishing Ki to the Organs, muscles, and limbs and up to the Heart
and Lungs as the basis for Ki and
Blood. Its warming, Yang Ki also
transforms body fluids. The Spleen
likes dryness, and hates damp. Cold
foods or too many cold drinks can
weaken the Spleen. Symptoms are
poor appetite and digestion, tiredness, weak muscles, heavy limbs,
watery stools or diarrhoea, and
swollen abdomen.

Spleen Ki also "holds the
Blood", preventing haemorrhage,
and "holds up" the Organs. Bruising, bleeding, haemorrhoids, varicose
veins, and all forms of prolapse are
symptoms of Spleen weakness.

CHANNEL EXERCISES

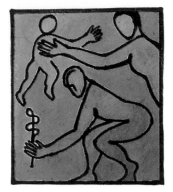

Stomach and Spleen

The following exercises help harmonize the Stomach and Spleen. Their Channels flow over the front of the body. The Spleen houses the intellect. Too much intellectual work or studying, especially when associated with irregular eating habits, can weaken the Spleen. In the same way, inability to concentrate, or poor memory, are symptoms of depleted Spleen. Exercise forms the ideal balance to intellectual work.

The sense of taste in the Five Element system is associated with the Spleen (see p. 25). The inability to taste food, or a dull, flat taste in the mouth indicate a Stomach-Spleen disharmony, as does craving for sweet foods – the specific flavour of the Earth Organs.

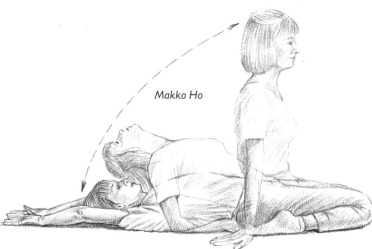

Makko Ho

From the seiza position (see p. 32), sit as low as you can between your heels. Do not proceed if your knees are painful but practise "just sitting" until you are comfortable.

Lean back on your hands, lifting and opening your chest. Then drop on to your elbows and finally all the way down (see left). Stretch your arms over your head if it is comfortable. Exhale as you move into each new position. Breathe 3 times in your final stretch. Move back through every stage slowly.

This yoga posture is an alternative stretch for people whose knees will not permit the stronger Makko Ho stretch. You can start this from an easy position, even sitting on a cushion between your heels.

Kneel up and bring your hands on to your heels to support your body. Lift your pelvis up and forward to arch your body on a full exhalation. Hold for a few breaths before coming out of the position.

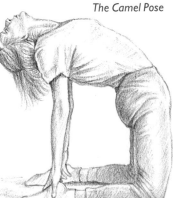

The Camel Pose

Stress and tension in the jaw

You may not think of the face as needing exercise, but it does. Stress and tension, often held unconsciously in the jaw muscle, may result in clenching and teeth grinding at night — a common problem.

The best exercise is to chew your food well, which benefits the Stomach directly. But you can also stretch, grimace, and move your jaw, and vocalize your feelings too. A more subtle, traditional exercise is to run your tongue around your gums to generate saliva — considered a precious fluid associated with the Spleen. Swallow and relax.

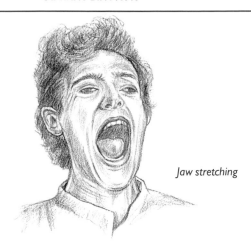

Jaw stretching

Releasing the solar plexus

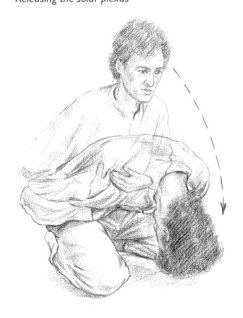

Tension in the diaphragm and stomach

The diaphragm, the stomach, and the solar plexus area are often held in tension, inhibiting breathing and circulation of Ki and Blood to the digestive Organs.

With your fingers turned in to the area just below your rib-cage, lean forward to apply gradually increasing pressure (see left). Always exhale slowly as you lean forward. Inhale as you sit up. Repeat a few times. The effect is purifying and invigorating.

Shiatsu routine for the front Channels

You can reach the Lung, Large Intestine, Stomach, and Spleen Channels most easily with your partner lying face up (the supine position).

Work on the Lung and Spleen Channels strengthens Ki and aids its circulation around the body. It warms the limbs and strengthens digestion. Bear in mind their specific functions (see pages 84 and 89) as you give shiatsu along these Channels.

The Large Intestine and Stomach Channels (see pages 85 and 88) meet on the face. Work on them can help in troubles of the eyes, nose, sinuses, teeth, and gums. The routine that follows on pages 92–103 starts with the arms, continues with the head and neck, and finishes on the legs.

Quiet preparation
Relax in seiza position by your partner's side and make contact by resting your palm on their Hara. Calm and centre yourself by taking note of how you feel and by acknowledging your condition. Pay attention to your partner's breathing. This is particularly important for your work on the Lung Channel.

Pick up your partner's arm with your outside hand and move your other hand from the Hara to clasp the top of your partner's shoulder. Lift the arm over your partner's head, then bring it round and down, out to the side. Repeat a few times (see also p. 50). Finally, place it on the floor at an angle of 45 degrees to your partner's side to start work on the Lung Channel.

Initial arm rotation

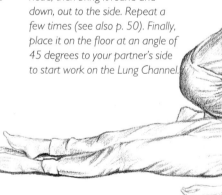

Lung Channel position

In order to lean comfortably and contact the Ki of the Lung Channel, move to the outside of the arm, facing in, with your partner's palm facing upward. Support your partner's shoulder with your nearside hand. Now lean *into the hollow area at the front of the shoulder (corresponding to points Lu 1 and Lu 2) and place your other hand anywhere along the arm (see left). Pause and relax, knees spread wide, before palming down the Channel.*

With your active hand locate the biceps muscle, and lean your weight through the line of your extended thumb and the heel of your palm into the space between the muscle and the humerus bone. Ease up, slide your hand along an inch or two, then relax and repeat the pressure. Continue in this way on the near side of the arm, palming down in easy stages to the wrist on the thumb side. Finish by gently squeezing along the sides of the thumb (see right).

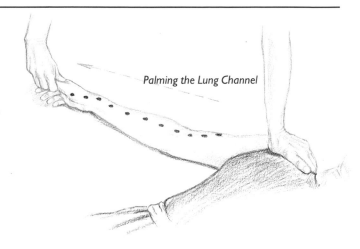

Palming the Lung Channel

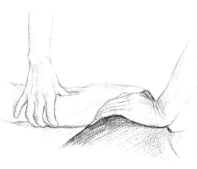

Investigating the groove

Now, with your fingers supporting the arm, use your extended thumb to explore the groove between the biceps muscle and the bone, for the tsubos. Slide your thumb along between these points, always keeping contact. Work into Lu 5 (see p. 84) on the outside of the biceps tendon at the elbow. Continue thumbing down the Channel, just inside the radius bone, toward Lu 9 at the base of the thumb (see p. 84). Pause to lean into the tsubos you find along the way.

Stay relaxed

Remember, keep your shoulders relaxed, extend your arms, and lean from your Hara. Don't squeeze or press with your thumb – it won't be effective and it may hurt.

Finish by grasping the base of your partner's thumb and squeezing firmly along its edges to the corners of the nail. Alternatively, thumb along the inside edge, including the "belly" of the muscle at the base of the thumb, where Lu 10 is found. This is a sedating point for painful sore throats.

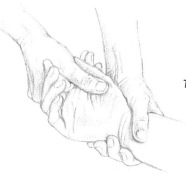

Thumbing the thumb at Lu 10

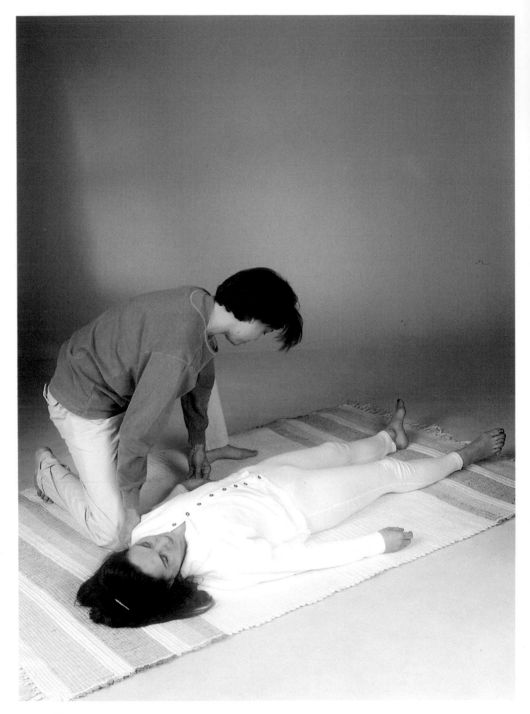

Thumbing the Large Intestine Channel

The Large Intestine Channel

You can work on this Channel with
very little adjustment to your position. All you need to do is rotate
your partner's hand slightly inward
(see below) to bring the edge of the
forearm uppermost. The Large Intestine Channel runs close to the Lung
Channel, but as it is Yang it is
nearer to the outside of the arm,
along the bony edge.

*Palming the Large Intestine
Channel*

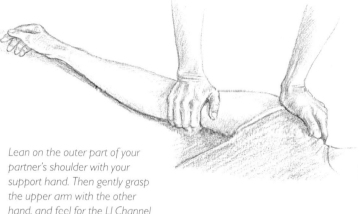

*Lean on the outer part of your
partner's shoulder with your
support hand. Then gently grasp
the upper arm with the other
hand, and feel for the LI Channel
along the humerus bone (see
above). Work with your flattened
thumb and heel of your palm.
Move your hand down in stages*

*past the elbow, leaning and gently
grasping, then along the bony
edge of the forearm.*

*When you are familiar with the
location of this Channel, try using
your thumb at a more penetrating
angle to work the upper arm (see
right). Work down to LI 11, at the
outside end of the elbow crease
when the arm is folded. Use this
point for feverish and hot
conditions, rashes, and itching.
Below the elbow use the Dragon's
Mouth technique (see p. 46) to
work down in stages from the
elbow to the wrist.*

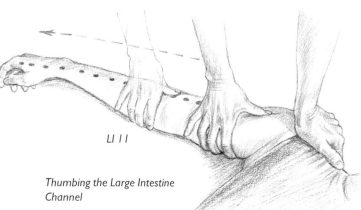

LI 11

*Thumbing the Large Intestine
Channel*

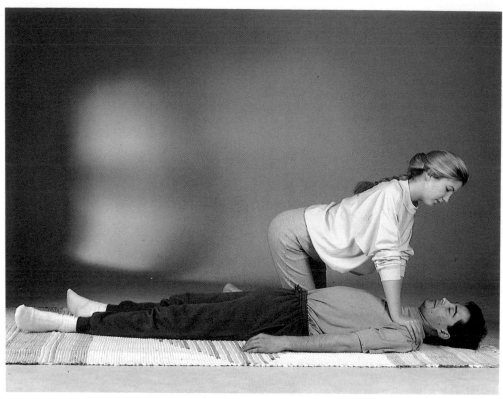

Leaning on the shoulders at Lung 1

Large Intestine 4

Find the high point of the muscle between the forefinger and thumb when closed. Then as your partner relaxes the muscle, press firmly down and toward the finger bone. This widely used point relieves aches and pains of the head, jaw, and teeth. It strengthens Yang and defensive Ki, and expels Wind, Cold, and Heat symptoms from the face, such as streaming colds, sneezing, sore eyes, and hay fever. Internally it has a strong, downward action that helps constipation and childbirth.

Caution Do not use this point during pregnancy.

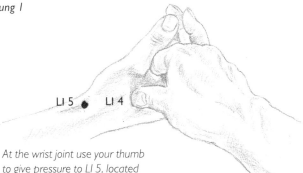

At the wrist joint use your thumb to give pressure to LI 5, located between the two tendons of the thumb. It is useful for pain in the wrist or thumb.

The LI Channel finishes on the forefinger. Grip or thumb along its edge to the nail and then pause for a moment when you finish, before quietly breaking contact and moving round to work on the Lung and LI Channels on the other side.

Working on the face and neck

Pause after finishing the arms, then keeping a light contact at your partner's shoulder if you can, move to a kneeling position with your knees spread wide either side of your partner's ears. Do not kneel too close as this will restrict your working circle, and may feel oppressive to your partner. Work on this area requires sensitivity. Approach the head and neck in a relaxed state of mind. Lean with both hands on your partner's shoulders and relax.

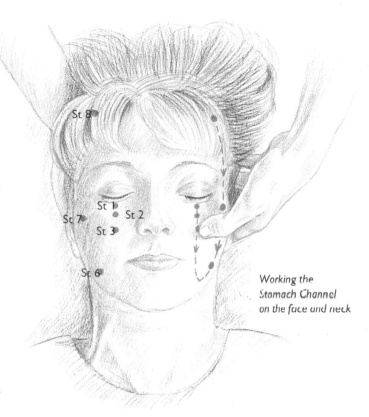

Working the Stomach Channel on the face and neck

Loosening the neck

Rest the palms of your hands loosely over the temples and ears for a few moments then, with your fingertips, hold the occipital ridge at the base of the skull behind the ears. Roll the head gently a few times from side to side to loosen the neck. Then, resting the edges of your hands on the floor, move your fingers farther under the head and curl them back into the hollows beneath the occipital bone. Lean back from the Hara to open and stretch the neck. This raises the back of your partner's head off the floor. Then slide your palms underneath so that the head rests comfortably in your hands. Keep your fingers where they are, cupping the back of the head — a pleasant sensation for your partner. Pause.

Roll your partner's head to the side, cradling and balancing it on the open palm and fingers of one hand. The other hand is now free to work the Stomach Channel along both its branches (see above) with the extended thumb. Begin at the point just inside the hairline at the corner of the forehead, St 8. The Channel passes down the side of the head, about 1 in (2 cm) in front of the ear. Feel for tsubos, including St 7 under the cheek bone and St 6 near the angle of the jaw in the middle of the powerful chewing muscle (Masseter muscle).

The other branch of this Channel begins on the border of the eye socket (the orbit) at St 1 and St 2. St 3 is under the cheek bone, level with the widest part of the nose. This point is good for sneezing and nasal troubles.

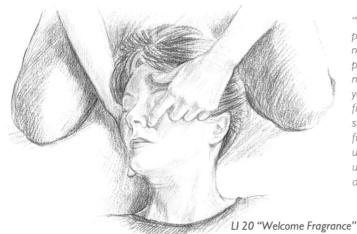

"Welcome Fragrance" is the last point of the LI Channel. As the name suggests, stimulating this point will help clear a sore, stuffy nose or sinuses. You may find that your index finger or even your little finger is better suited to stimulating LI 20. Extend the finger and lean at a slight angle upward and in toward the nose using the weight of your relaxed arm (see left).

LI 20 "Welcome Fragrance"

Still cradling the head at a slight angle, work down the prominent muscle at the side of the neck (sterno-cleido-mastoid). The LI Channel runs along its top, and the Stomach Channel a little to the front. Rest the ball of your thumb over the muscle, the fingers of your working hand supporting the back of your partner's neck. Try to feel as if your two hands are cooperating and connected (see p. 52). Alter the attitude of your partner's head a little to promote relaxation as you work down both Channels on the muscle.

Work on the other side
Replace the working hand under the skull to match the position of the other one, before rolling the head over gently to repeat the work on Stomach and Large Intestine Channels on the other side of the face.

Working the neck

Lifting the neck and stretching the spine

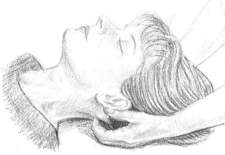

Return your partner's head to its natural position, move your hands down and overlap your fingers to encircle the underside of the neck below the skull. Keep your thumbs tucked positively against your partner's jawbone. Lift up and back, gently arching the neck and, by sinking back from your hips, give a little stretch to the spine.

Replace the head on the ground in a comfortable position, pulling back slightly on the occipital ridge under the skull.

Finish this routine as you began, leaning on to your partner's shoulders. Gently break contact after a few moments.

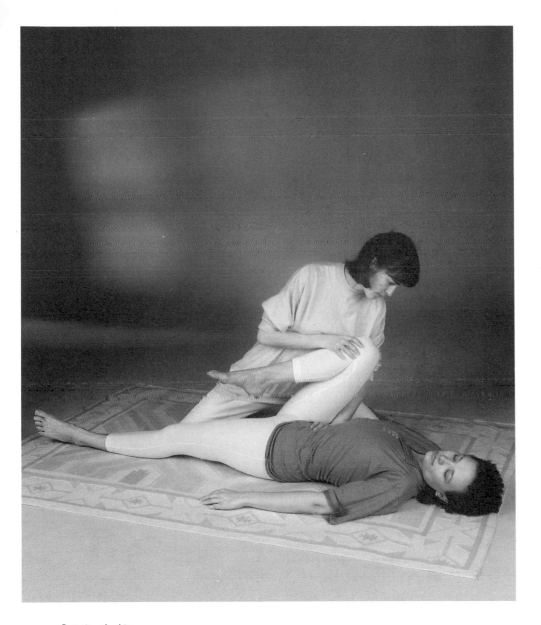

Rotating the hip

Positioning for the Leg Channels
The Stomach and Spleen Channels
descend the front of the thigh and
leg. The Stomach Channel, being
Yang, runs outside the Yin Spleen
Channel (see pp. 88–9). The
Stomach and Spleen govern digestion
and belong to the Earth element.
Work on their Channels in the leg
will connect your partner "ener-
getically" with the Earth (see p.
22) and strengthen digestion. Kneel
facing your partner, your knees
spread wide.

*Place one hand below the navel;
the other, fingers pointing out, on
top of your partner's thigh. Palm
down in stages to the knee,
turning your fingers inward once
you are below the level of the
groin. Then try the Stomach
Channel stretch (below).*

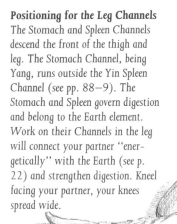

*Palming the
Stomach Channel*

*Roll your partner's near leg inward
and extend your own leg to rest
the sole of your foot, heel on the
ground, across the front of your
partner's foot. This brings the
Stomach Channel uppermost.
Then kneel up, bring your hips
forward, and palm the Channel
again, this time from the upper
thigh to the lower leg. The stretch
activates the Ki in the Channel. It
may seem difficult, but try it.*

*Stretching the
Stomach Channel*

*From the same position thumb the
Stomach Channel down the leg.
Slide your thumb between tsubos
to St 34, 2in (5cm) above the
kneecap. Continue over the knee
to St 36 – one hand's breadth
below the kneecap (see right and
p. 101), and down the leg,
following the Stomach Channel
about one finger-width outside
the shinbone.*

*Thumbing the
Stomach
Channel*

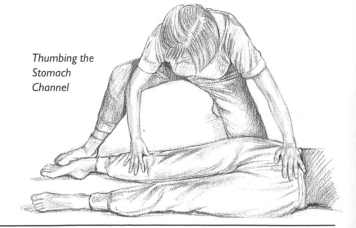

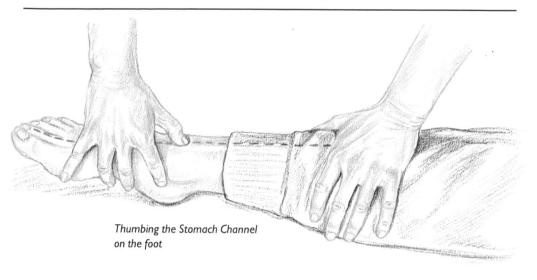

Thumbing the Stomach Channel
on the foot

Stomach 36 ("Leg Three Miles")

Ancient physicians said that any
disease could be treated by this
point. It can be used to strengthen
and tonify the whole system safely.
St 36 works on the Stomach and the
Spleen, which according to traditional Oriental medicine extract
Blood and Ki from food. It is said
that Chinese foot soldiers used to
halt every three miles and massage
St 36 for renewed energy – hence its
name. Soldiers of the revolutionary
peasant army who followed Mao Tse
Tung on the incredible "Long
March" across China, 1934–5,
are reported to have done the same.

*As you reach the foot, bring your
supporting hand down from the
Hara to any part of the leg, above
or below the knee, or even to the
ankle. Thumb over the highest
part of the foot (see above) to
St 44 between the 2nd and 3rd
toes (see below). Work into St 44,
then to the end of the Channel on
the outside of the second toe;
squeeze it firmly and stretch it.*

Stomach 44 ("Inner Courtyard")

Half an inch (1cm) before the web
between the second and third toes is
St 44. To find this point press
toward the bone of the second toe.
Work on St 44 to alleviate stomach
ache or acidity; for acute problems
work on St 36 and St 34 as well.
St 44 will also help relieve toothache, sore or bleeding gums, redness
and irritation of the eyes, or frontal
headaches. For problems of the face
or mouth also work on the Large
Intestine Channel, especially
LI 4 (see p. 96).

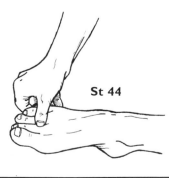

St 44

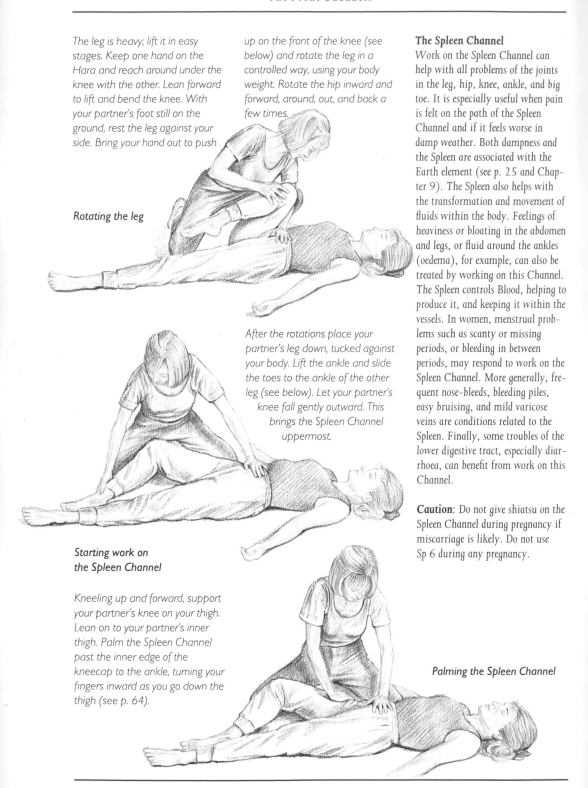

The leg is heavy; lift it in easy stages. Keep one hand on the Hara and reach around under the knee with the other. Lean forward to lift and bend the knee. With your partner's foot still on the ground, rest the leg against your side. Bring your hand out to push up on the front of the knee (see below) and rotate the leg in a controlled way, using your body weight. Rotate the hip inward and forward, around, out, and back a few times.

Rotating the leg

After the rotations place your partner's leg down, tucked against your body. Lift the ankle and slide the toes to the ankle of the other leg (see below). Let your partner's knee fall gently outward. This brings the Spleen Channel uppermost.

Starting work on the Spleen Channel

Kneeling up and forward, support your partner's knee on your thigh. Lean on to your partner's inner thigh. Palm the Spleen Channel past the inner edge of the kneecap to the ankle, turning your fingers inward as you go down the thigh (see p. 64).

Palming the Spleen Channel

The Spleen Channel

Work on the Spleen Channel can help with all problems of the joints in the leg, hip, knee, ankle, and big toe. It is especially useful when pain is felt on the path of the Spleen Channel and if it feels worse in damp weather. Both dampness and the Spleen are associated with the Earth element (see p. 25 and Chapter 9). The Spleen also helps with the transformation and movement of fluids within the body. Feelings of heaviness or bloating in the abdomen and legs, or fluid around the ankles (oedema), for example, can also be treated by working on this Channel. The Spleen controls Blood, helping to produce it, and keeping it within the vessels. In women, menstrual problems such as scanty or missing periods, or bleeding in between periods, may respond to work on the Spleen Channel. More generally, frequent nose-bleeds, bleeding piles, easy bruising, and mild varicose veins are conditions related to the Spleen. Finally, some troubles of the lower digestive tract, especially diarrhoea, can benefit from work on this Channel.

Caution: Do not give shiatsu on the Spleen Channel during pregnancy if miscarriage is likely. Do not use Sp 6 during any pregnancy.

After palming, the tsubos on the Spleen Channel will be easier to find. The classical points, Sp 10, 9, 6, and 3, described below, are useful to know and act as landmarks on the way. Slide your thumb lightly along the Channel, working into receptive points. The inner leg can be tender: move from your Hara to increase pressure gradually (see p. 53).

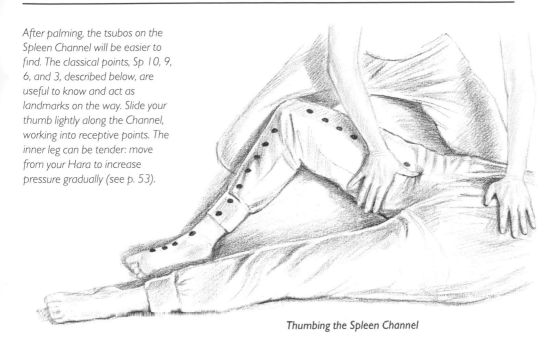

Thumbing the Spleen Channel

Spleen 3 ("Greater Whiteness")

This point is just behind the prominent joint of the big toe on the side of the foot, slightly beneath the bone. Its name suggests a pallid complexion associated with weak Blood. Spleen 3 strengthens the Spleen and helps when weak digestion is combined with poor appetite, when bowel motions are loose, or if there is colonic bleeding. This point helps poor memory, muddled thinking, or mental fatigue. It also strengthens the neck and spine.

Spleen 6 ("Three Yin Meeting")

Spleen 6 is found one hand's breadth up from the inside ankle bone, in the hollow in the muscle just behind the bone. The three Yin Channels of the Spleen, Liver, and Kidneys meet here. Generally, Sp 6 strengthens and regulates Blood. It is used in all male and female sexual problems — impotence, infertility, menstrual irregularities, period pains, and discharges. In women it influences the uterus, promoting contractions during childbirth and easing labour pains (see Chapter 10).
Caution: Do not use Sp 6 during pregnancy.

Spleen 9 ("Yin Mountain Pond")

This point is about 2 in (5cm) below the knee on the inside, in the hollow between the head of the large bone (the tibia) and the calf muscle. It helps the Spleen to control fluids and is useful for pains in the knee, especially those made worse by damp, and when stiffness increases with lack of movement, for example, in bed or sitting still.

Spleen 10 ("Sea of Blood")

Just 2 in (5cm) above the kneecap on its inner edge, in the height of the muscular bulge, is Sp 10. The point is useful to control bleeding in people who have a tendency toward mild haemorrhages. It has a cooling action on the Blood and will ease hot rashes and itching.

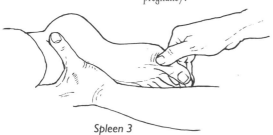

Spleen 3

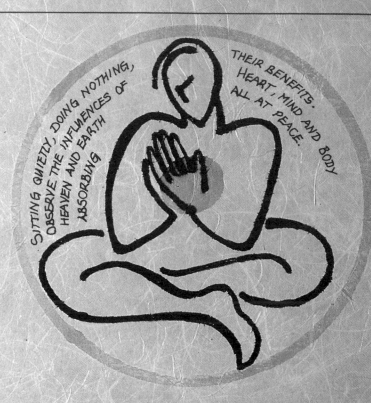

SITTING QUIETLY, DOING NOTHING, OBSERVE THE INFLUENCES OF HEAVEN AND EARTH ABSORBING THEIR BENEFITS. HEART, MIND AND BODY ALL AT PEACE.

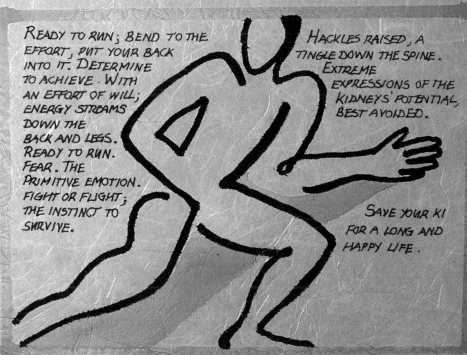

READY TO RUN; BEND TO THE EFFORT, PUT YOUR BACK INTO IT. DETERMINE TO ACHIEVE. WITH AN EFFORT OF WILL; ENERGY STREAMS DOWN THE BACK AND LEGS. READY TO RUN. FEAR. THE PRIMITIVE EMOTION. FIGHT OR FLIGHT; THE INSTINCT TO SURVIVE.

HACKLES RAISED, A TINGLE DOWN THE SPINE. EXTREME EXPRESSIONS OF THE KIDNEYS' POTENTIAL, BEST AVOIDED.

SAVE YOUR KI FOR A LONG AND HAPPY LIFE.

CHAPTER SEVEN

The Back Channels

HEART · SMALL INTESTINE
BLADDER · KIDNEY

The Heart, deep and hidden, is the Organ of central control, the seat of consciousness and "House of the Mind"; the centre of response to the emotional environment. It governs Blood and controls blood vessels and circulation. Blood not only nourishes the physical body but embraces and supports the Mind. Like the emperor of old, performing sacred rites to harmonize the elements and ensure peace and prosperity among the people, when the Heart performs well the body flourishes and the Mind is serene and happy. Those people who have a strong constitution, a lively mind, a sparkle in their eyes, and an open, warm, and sensible disposition reflect the work of this Organ. The Small Intestine assists the Heart in its capacity to discern ideas, clarify thoughts, and absorb shock.

The Kidneys are more basic. They are called the "Root of Life". All organisms are impelled by the need to survive; to protect themselves and reproduce. The impetus of these drives manifests through the Kidneys. Assisted by the Bladder, they control purification, reserves, efficient hormonal and nervous systems, preparedness, and power to take action. The Kidneys are the foundation of Yin and Yang. They store constitutional Essence, and govern birth, growth, and reproduction.

In Five Element terms, Heart and Small Intestine (see top, facing page) belong to Fire, the uprising tendency, summer, heat, the colour red, the sound of laughter, and the emotion of joy or happiness. By contrast the Bladder and Kidneys (see bottom, facing page) belong to Water, the sinking, collecting tendency, winter, cold, the colour blue-black, the groaning sound, and the emotion of fear.

You can work on all four Channels with your partner lying face down - the prone position. Follow the pathway details for these Channels on pages 106-7 and 110-11, the Channel exercises on pages 108 and 112-13, and the routine for the four Channels (on pages 114-27).

The Heart Channel pathway

This Channel begins in the Heart and emerges via the surrounding blood vessels to pass down through the diaphragm to the Small Intestine, its related Organ. Another internal branch ascends through the throat to the eye, and a connecting Channel goes to the tongue.

A third branch goes first to the Lung before surfacing at the centre of the armpit. From here the Channel descends along the inner aspect of the arm, on the opposite side of the biceps to the Lung Channel, passing the inner end of the elbow crease. It continues down to the tip of the little finger by the corner of the nail on the thumbside.

When giving shiatsu in the supine position it is best to fold the arm into the Heart Channel stretch position (see right), which makes it easily accessible. For shiatsu in the prone position, as in this chapter, work with the arm away from the side, palm turned up.

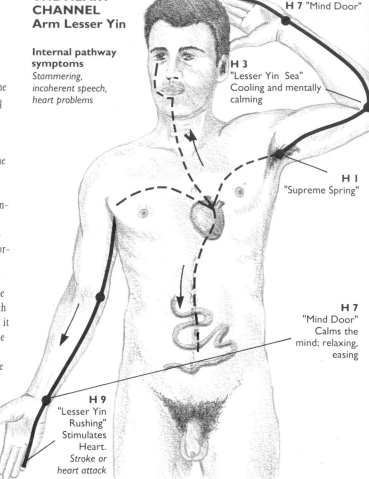

THE HEART CHANNEL
Arm Lesser Yin

Internal pathway symptoms
Stammering, incoherent speech, heart problems

H 7 "Mind Door"

H 3 "Lesser Yin Sea" Cooling and mentally calming

H 1 "Supreme Spring"

H 7 "Mind Door" Calms the mind; relaxing, easing

H 9 "Lesser Yin Rushing" Stimulates Heart. *Stroke or heart attack*

The Heart Channel – functions and associated symptoms

Constitutional strength depends on the Heart as well as the Kidneys (see p. 105). Accordingly, disorders of the Heart may result in weakness, tiredness, or lethargy, and sometimes in dizziness or palpitations. The close relationship of Blood and Ki means that the Lungs may be affected as well, resulting in breathlessness (see p. 84).

The Heart belongs to the Fire element, moves Blood, and houses the Mind. The Channel opens

to the tongue and controls sweat.

Heart disharmonies are often characterized by disorders of the circulation, such as stuffiness or pains in the chest, and feeling too hot or too cold, especially in the hands. Imbalance in the Heart may also produce mental and emotional disorders such as restlessness, insomnia, or dream-disturbed sleep, and nervousness, irritability, or anxiety. Abnormal sweating may accompany any of these symptoms.

The face colour reflects the state of the circulation and, therefore, of the Heart (see pp. 160–1). A pale, lifeless complexion suggests weakness of Heart Ki or Blood; a red complexion indicates that Heat is affecting the Heart.

Heart disharmonies show themselves in the tongue, producing speech difficulties, such as stammering. Many talkative, excitable, overjolly people may be manifesting a Heart imbalance.

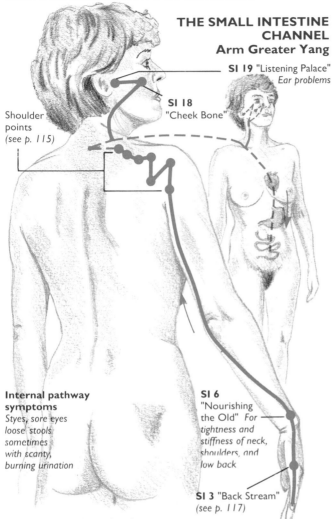

THE SMALL INTESTINE CHANNEL
Arm Greater Yang

SI 19 "Listening Palace"
Ear problems

SI 18
"Cheek Bone"

Shoulder
points
(see p. 115)

**Internal pathway
symptoms**
*Styes, sore eyes
loose stools
sometimes
with scanty,
burning urination*

SI 6
"Nourishing
the Old" *For
tightness and
stiffness of neck,
shoulders, and
low back*

SI 3 "Back Stream"
(see p. 117)

The Small Intestine Channel pathway

This Channel starts on the other corner of the little fingernail from the Heart Channel (see page opposite) and follows the edge of the hand to the wrist, where it turns slightly to flow up the forearm, close to the outer edge of the (ulna) bone. Passing the elbow at the "funny bone", it continues up the back of the arm, behind the shoulder joint. It then curves across the shoulder blade to connect with the Governing Vessel at GV 14 as do all Yang Channels. It crosses forward to the hollow above the collarbone where the internal branch penetrates, first to the Heart, then along the oesophagus to the Stomach, before connecting with its own Organ, the Small Intestine.

From the collarbone region the superficial path continues up behind the muscle on the side of the neck (sterno-cleido-mastoid), then over the cheek to the ear. Two internal branches separate on the cheek. They lead to the Gall Bladder Channel on the outer corner of the eye, and to the Bladder Channel — the next in the cycle (see p. 79) — at Bl 1 on the inner corner.

The Small Intestine — functions and associated symptoms

The Small Intestine receives partially transformed food and drink from the Stomach and separates and absorbs the nourishing part for the Spleen to distribute. It moves the solid waste to the Large Intestine, passing "impure fluids" to the Bladder. The role of this Channel can be summarized as receiving, separating, assimilating, and transforming.

The Small Intestine is linked with the Heart, and helps it to give clarity to the Mind, discerning

and absorbing good ideas. Muddled thinking is a sign of weakness in the Small Intestine.

The role of separating and transforming fluids is shared with the Bladder. Both Organs are located in the lower region of the body, controlled by the Kidneys. Because of the Bladder connections, work on the Small Intestine Channel helps to relieve posterior headaches and pain in the spine and lower back. Frequent and profuse, or scanty, burn-

ing urination may be treated by work on these three Channels.

Channel symptoms of the Small Intestine include pain and stiffness of the wrist, elbow, or shoulder blade area and neck, earache, and sore, red eyes.

CHANNEL EXERCISES

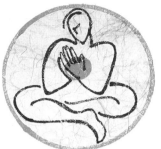

Heart and Small Intestine

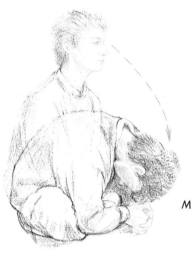

Stress, poor diet, and over-eating are now recognized as the main causes of circulation and heart troubles. If you are too rushed to choose foods wisely and too stressed to eat and digest comfortably, you will weaken your constitution and jeopardize your heart.

The Heart Channel goes to the tongue and helps the Spleen to distinguish the "five flavours" and so choose appropriate foods. The Small Intestine supports the Stomach and Spleen in digestion, as well as assisting your judgement in all matters.

The Heart and Small Intestine Makko Ho exercise derives from the posture of prayer and meditation. The stretch gently activates both Channels by opening the neck and shoulders, which stimulates the course of Ki in the Channels in the arm. It also opens and invigorates the chest and abdominal cavities where the Organs are located. The simple message behind these exercises is – eat less and relax more.

Sit with your knees bent and the soles of your feet together. Clasp your feet, bringing them as close to your groin as comfortable. Let your knees drop. Then, using your feet as an anchor, lift open your chest and exhaling slowly, fold forward from this position until the end of the breath. Relax in the furthest position, elbows outside the knees, breathing several times into your Hara. Inhale as you sit up.

Makko Ho stretch

Empty the Heart
of everything,
let the Mind be
at peace
LAO TZU
TAO TE CHING

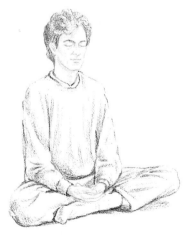

Meditation pose

It is not so much the formal posture that is important – more the inner practice. Sit or kneel in any position with your spine relaxed and upright. Use a cushion or sit in a chair if you like. Relax your hands, close your eyes, and spend up to 15 minutes just being aware of your breath or listening to its sound. You will be distracted, but do not worry; just start again. There is nothing to achieve; nowhere to go.

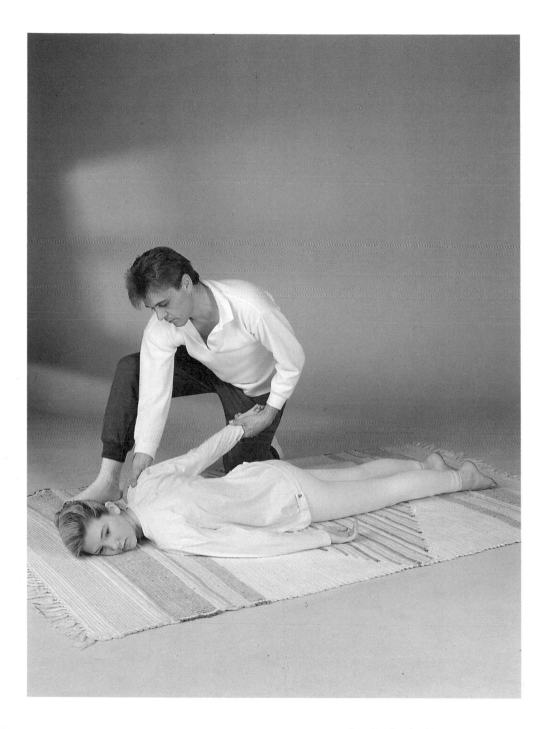

Rotating the shoulder

The Bladder Channel pathway

The Bladder Channel begins at the inner corner of the eye, rising up through the eyebrow (Bl 2) over the forehead and skull to join the Governing Vessel at GV 20. Here it enters the brain, re-emerging as a superficial path at the nape of the neck. This path continues over the base of the skull (occiput), where it divides again into two branches that descend parallel with the spine. The inner branch diverts briefly to meet GV 14 before continuing to the sacrum, then on down the back of the thigh to the centre of the knee-fold. An internal branch connects with the Kidney and then the Bladder, after separating at the lumbar region. The outer branch passes from the occiput along the edge of the shoulder blade and descends to the buttock, continuing down the thigh to meet the other branch at the knee. The single Channel continues down the centre of the calf muscle and passes behind the outer ankle to the outer tip of the little toe.

The Bladder Channel – functions and associated symptoms

The Bladder transforms waste fluids into urine, which it then excretes, helping the Kidneys to regulate water. But its Channel has a wider influence. It is an aspect of Kidney Yang, which helps in defence and supports other Organs via the associated points (see p. 123). The Kidneys "nourish the brain and spinal cord". The Bladder Channel connects with the brain and helps integrate intelligence with the functions of the nervous system.

Bladder disharmony can manifest as mental symptoms — jealousy, suspicion, obsessions, restlessness, and strained nerves.

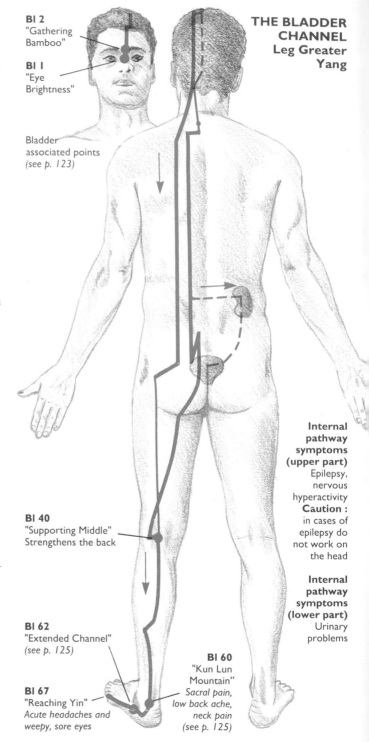

Bl 2
"Gathering Bamboo"

Bl 1
"Eye Brightness"

Bladder associated points (see p. 123)

**THE BLADDER CHANNEL
Leg Greater Yang**

Bl 40
"Supporting Middle"
Strengthens the back

Bl 62
"Extended Channel"
(see p. 125)

Bl 67
"Reaching Yin"
Acute headaches and weepy, sore eyes

Bl 60
"Kun Lun Mountain"
Sacral pain, low back ache, neck pain
(see p. 125)

Internal pathway symptoms (upper part)
Epilepsy, nervous hyperactivity
Caution :
in cases of epilepsy do not work on the head

Internal pathway symptoms (lower part)
Urinary problems

THE KIDNEY CHANNEL
Leg Lesser Yin

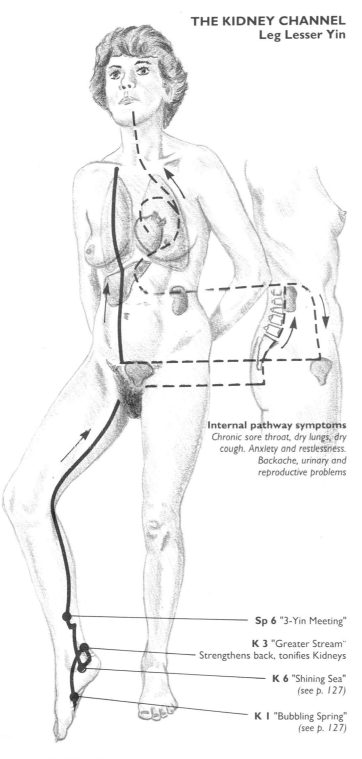

Internal pathway symptoms
Chronic sore throat, dry lungs, dry cough. Anxiety and restlessness. Backache, urinary and reproductive problems

Sp 6 "3-Yin Meeting"

K 3 "Greater Stream"
Strengthens back, tonifies Kidneys

K 6 "Shining Sea"
(see p. 127)

K 1 "Bubbling Spring"
(see p. 127)

The Kidney Channel pathway

This Channel begins under the little toe, near the end of the Bladder Channel, and crosses through K 1 to the inner edge of the foot. It loops behind the inside ankle bone to the heel, then rises along the inner aspect of the leg, intersecting the Spleen Channel at Sp 6, before continuing up the calf and the inner thigh.

Here its pathway becomes deeper and goes to the base of the spine, where it joins the Governing Vessel. Rising internally in line with the lumbar spine it enters the Kidney, descends to the Bladder, and surfaces at the pubic area. It connects with the Directing Vessel in the lower abdomen and then rises over the body to the collarbone.

Internally a branch leaves the Kidney to enter the Liver and Lung, and continues up to the throat and tongue. From the Lung another branch flows to the Heart and chest, and joins the Pericardium Channel.

The Kidneys — functions and associated symptoms

The Kidneys are the basis of our constitutional strength and control energy and substance in the body. They also rule the bones, open to the ear, and manifest in the head hair. Kidney Yin stores Essence, the basis of physical growth, development, and maturity. It forms "Marrow" for the brain and spinal cord, as well as bone marrow.

Kidney Yang is the body's "transforming power" and supports the functions of all other Organs.

Kidney symptoms are characterized by weakness and depletion and commonly include urinary and sexual problems, sore, aching lower back, poor memory, dizziness, hearing loss, ringing in the ears, and thinning or loss of hair.

CHANNEL EXERCISES

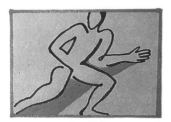

Bladder and Kidneys

The role of the Bladder and Kidney in supporting the body can lead to depletion. Excessive mental work can lead to brain fatigue, irritability, insomnia, and inability to relax. Excessive physical work can deplete both Ki and Essence, producing many symptoms (see p. 111). It is also important to regulate sexual activity to suit your energies, as the combination of overwork with excessive sex can provoke more serious Kidney disharmonies. The Makko Ho stretch (below) rejuvenates and relaxes your body. Do it before sleeping.

Exercise is important to balance the use of mental energy, but rest and relaxation is equally necessary to balance physical work. Balance physical work with restful pleasures.

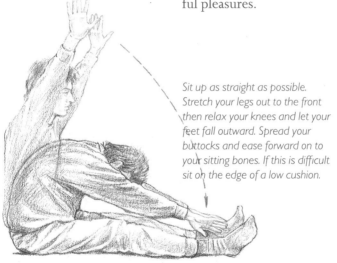

Sit up as straight as possible. Stretch your legs out to the front then relax your knees and let your feet fall outward. Spread your buttocks and ease forward on to your sitting bones. If this is difficult sit on the edge of a low cushion.

Inhale and raise your arms straight above your head, palms outward. Then fold forward from your hips, keeping your chest and back extended, and exhaling as you bend. Bring your hands toward your feet, but do not try to grip your legs or pull down. Just stay in the forward bend and breathe; relax your back, neck, shoulders, arms, and legs.

Remain in this position for a minute or two if you are comfortable.

Makko Ho stretches

This simple waist rotation loosens the waist and stretches the back so helping the flow of Ki up and down all the Channels. It brings direct benefit to a tired, aching, sore back – a common Kidney deficiency complaint.

Stand with your feet wide apart and parallel, knees bent. Support your back behind your waist or under the back ribs. Keeping your hips and legs still, turn at the waist to face 45 degrees to one side, then fold forward over one knee and look down. Circle smoothly across to the other knee. Lift your head and chest and face the front. Repeat the rotations for a few minutes, exhaling slowly as you bend forward and inhaling as you come up. Then change direction.

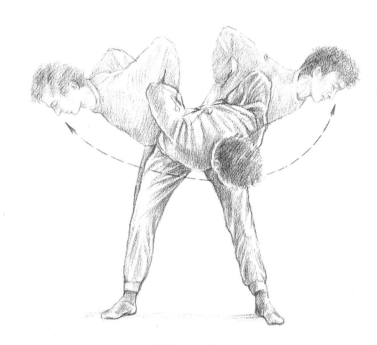

Waist rotations

Warming the Kidneys

Rubbing is a natural, spontaneous way of stimulating and attracting Ki. It has long been included in traditional exercise systems.

Stand with your feet a shoulder-width apart, knees relaxed. Rub your hands together for a minute, holding them in front of your chest. Try to keep your shoulders relaxed. Breathe deeply. When your hands are warm, place them on your back over the Kidney area. Lean forward slightly and rub vigorously. Inhale through your mouth and blow as you exhale. Repeat once or twice. Combine this with the exercises for the Lungs (p. 86) and Triple Burner (p. 135) on cold mornings.

Shiatsu routine for the back Channels

These four Channels flow on the inner posterior surfaces of the body and limbs and so are most easily treated with your partner lying face down.

The Heart and Small Intestine Channels on the arm, and the Bladder and Kidney Channels on the leg, represent Fire and Water, which, when in harmony, uphold and maintain constitutional strength. The Heart and Kidneys give each other mutual support. The Small Intestine and Bladder cooperate in transforming fluids and both their Channels influence the head, the neck, and the whole spine.

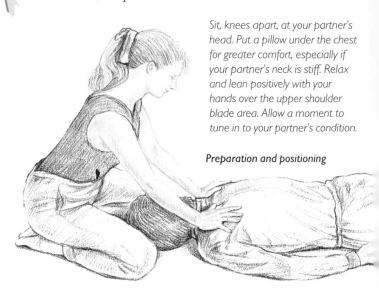

Sit, knees apart, at your partner's head. Put a pillow under the chest for greater comfort, especially if your partner's neck is stiff. Relax and lean positively with your hands over the upper shoulder blade area. Allow a moment to tune in to your partner's condition.

Preparation and positioning

Thumbing the Small Intestine Channel

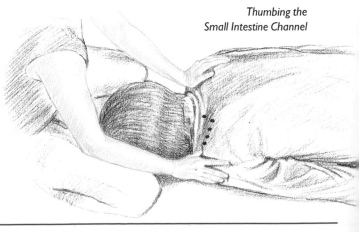

Thumb along the SI Channel from the base of the neck to the shoulder extremity twice each side. Place your support hand on the opposite shoulder. The line runs across the top of the shoulder blade to the hollow point at the end. The Channel also runs down on to the shoulder blade; work into any tsubos you find.

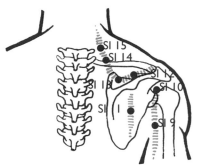

Points for the neck and shoulder

Local points
The classical points SI 15, 14, 13, 12, and 11 (in the order of working), and SI 9 and 10 in the arm space above the arm pit crease where arm and shoulder join, are locally effective points for problems of the neck and shoulder region.

Work one side at a time, leaning with the "knife-edge" of your hand into the muscle area between the shoulder and the bone of the arm – SI 9 and 10. Use your fingers or thumbs for deeper penetration but try using the edge of the hand first: it is very effective and feels more friendly – especially important when the shoulders are stiff.

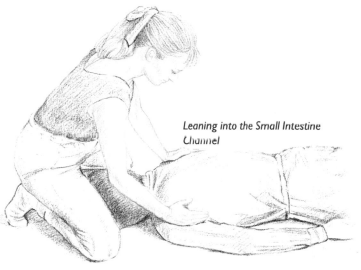

Leaning into the Small Intestine Channel

Thumbing the Bladder Channel on the shoulders

Palm the general area between the shoulder blades, each side of the spine. Use one hand at a time or both together. Then thumb along the inner line of the Bladder Channel – the ridge of muscles about 1.5 in (3 cm) from the mid line. Work down as far as the tip of the shoulder blades, then return and give pressure along the outer line of the Channel 3in (7cm) from the mid line. Bring your weight forward as you work down..

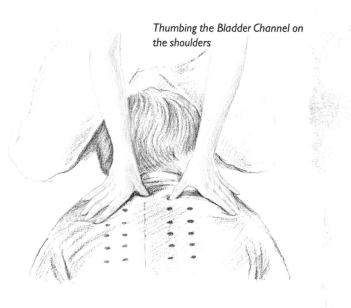

The Small Intestine Channel on the arm

As you work down the Small Intestine Channel of the arm to the fingers, the range of its influence increases. Symptoms such as headaches, sore, red eyes, acute earache, or acute gastric or urinary troubles can be eased by shiatsu along this Channel. The tsubos along the forearm to the fingers connect with other Channels, producing a calming effect on the Heart and Mind. The Bladder Channel is also affected, relaxing the spine and lower back.

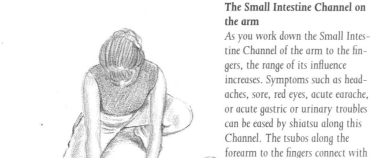

Palming the Small Intestine Channel

Move to your partner's side, and remain in contact as you do so. Lift your partner's wrist, move the arm out a little and on to its edge to bring the little finger uppermost.

Palm the arm from the shoulder area above the armpit down to the wrist. Relax your fingers around the arm and steady it with a gentle grip as you explore its contours.

Dragon's Mouth

This technique (see p. 46) is useful for working the SI Channel in the upper arm after palming. The Channel can be awkward to thumb from your position on the outside, but the bottom knuckle of your forefinger will find it naturally. Apply pressure on each tsubo.

Begin thumbing at SI 8 (see left and top p. 117) between the elbow's bony point and the rounded tip of bone on the inner aspect of the joint. Then, move to the outer edge of the forearm (ulna) (see centre p. 117). After the raised prominence above the wrist, follow the Channel across the edge of the hand.

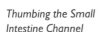

Thumbing the Small Intestine Channel

Following the Channels

Following the pathways of any arm Channel, especially the Yang Channels, can be bewildering as they can appear to deviate sharply at the elbow from one aspect to another. The Small Intestine Channel does just this. Nevertheless it is easy to reach on both upper and lower parts of the arm when your partner is lying in the prone position. The Dragon's Mouth technique is particularly suitable on the upper arm but the thumb works best below the elbow. Sit back a little to work along the outer aspect of the bone. At the wrist you will need to change position again, moving up and for ward to lean down along the edge of the hand. Finish at the little finger.

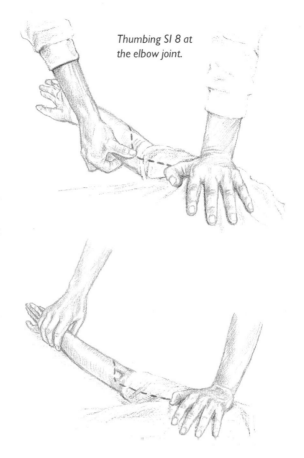

Thumbing SI 8 at the elbow joint.

Thumbing the Small Intestine Channel on the forearm.

Small Intestine 3

The Small Intestine Channel runs between the muscle and the bone along the border between the paler and darker skin on the outer edge of the hand. SI 3 has a particularly wide influence and is situated on this line just before the knuckle of the little finger, at the tip of the crease made by folding the hand.

This point works through its own Channel, and via connections with the Bladder Channel and Governing Vessel. It strengthens the spine, relaxes muscles and tendons, calms the Mind, and helps clear judgement and decision-making.

It is useful after shock or injury affecting the neck and spine, such as whiplash; also for feverish chills with shivers and spasms; for stiffness in the neck or spine, painful red eyes, ear troubles, dizziness, posterior headaches, pain in the fingers or arm, and pain or stiffness across the lower back.

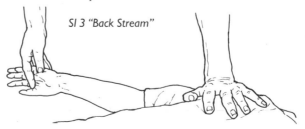

SI 3 "Back Stream"

Treating the Heart Channel

Physical and emotional stress upset the Heart. Cold hands and feet, lethargy, spontaneous sweating, and a shiny, pale face are signs that the Heart Ki is weak. Restless, dream-disturbed sleep, hot sweaty palms, flushed cheeks, dizziness, nervousness, and irritability show that Fire and Water are unbalanced, weakening the Blood. Shiatsu for the Heart Channel can have a deeply calming effect and benefit circulation.

Positioning for the Heart Channel

The position for working on the Heart Channel is shown on the facing page. Place your support hand on the heart area of the back between the shoulder blades. By turning your partner's hand so the palm is facing up you will expose the inner aspect of the arm, where the Channel runs.

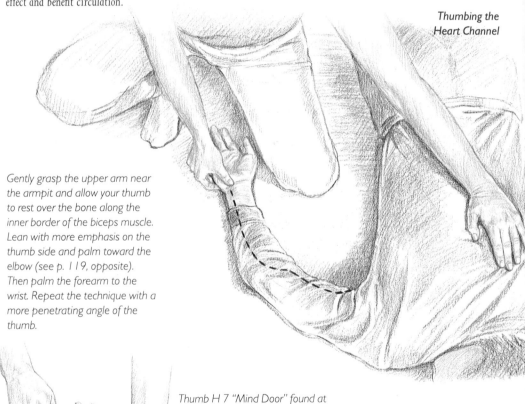

Thumbing the Heart Channel

Gently grasp the upper arm near the armpit and allow your thumb to rest over the bone along the inner border of the biceps muscle. Lean with more emphasis on the thumb side and palm toward the elbow (see p. 119, opposite). Then palm the forearm to the wrist. Repeat the technique with a more penetrating angle of the thumb.

Squeezing the finger

H 7

Thumb H 7 "Mind Door" found at the wrist crease (see left). This point is well known for its calming but supportive effect on the Heart and Mind.

Finish by thumbing across the palm to the little finger, then gently squeeze along both sides of the finger to its tip (see left).

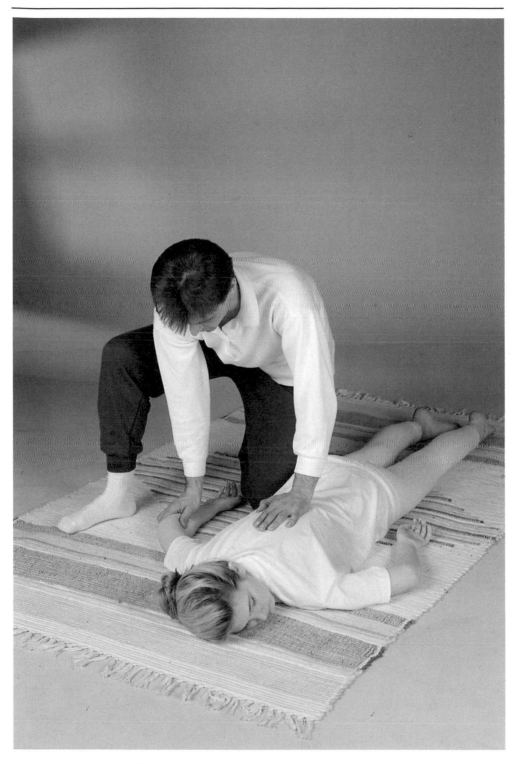

Palming the Heart Channel

Rotating the limbs

Lifting and moving limbs can be hard work. But it is easy to do if you use your body to follow through the movement, keep your shoulders and elbows relaxed, and take support wherever possible – for example from your raised leg (see below).

Pick up your partner's arm by the wrist with your nearside hand. Scoop your outside hand under the shoulder. Lean back slightly to stretch out the shoulder, then lift it and push it in over the ribs, then up toward the neck. Release and stretch back to begin again. Repeat 3 or 4 times. After the rotation try the shoulder slash technique (below). If the shoulders seem tight just thumb round the inner border of the shoulder blade.

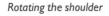

Rotating the shoulder

To "slash" the shoulder place your partner's hand on to their back. Ask your partner to "let go" both elbow and shoulder. Cup the outer shoulder with one hand and place the index finger of the other firmly alongside the shoulder blade border. Lift with the outer hand; lean in with the other, inserting the fingers positively under the blade for a moment. Release and repeat several times.

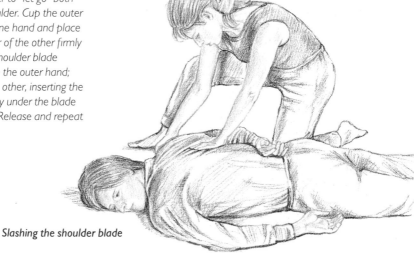

Slashing the shoulder blade

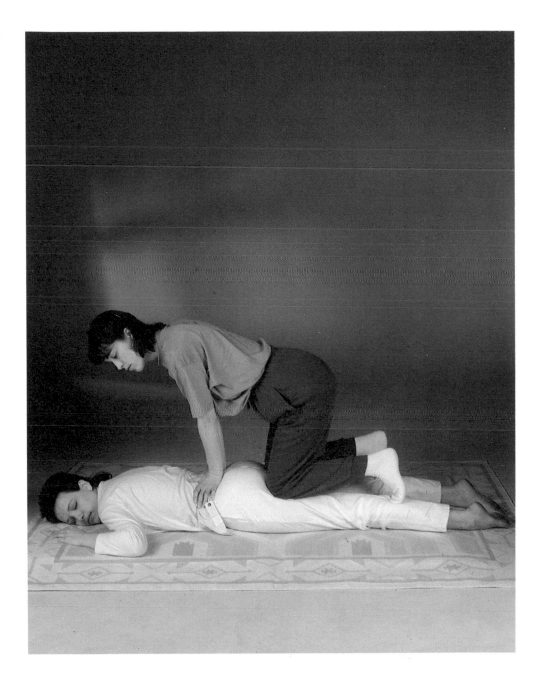

Distributing the body weight – strong but safe work on the Bladder Channel.

The Bladder Channel

Work on this Channel benefits the back, releases tension, and tonifies the Bladder and Kidneys. It also nourishes the other Organs via the "associated points" (see facing page). Treating the lumbar and sacral areas is good for sexual and menstrual problems and can often relieve period and labour pains. Work on the leg is useful for acute back troubles and haemorrhoids, and tsubos on the foot will particularly affect the eyes, nose, neck, and head.

After working on the shoulder, turn in to face your partner. Work down the Bladder Channel using your palm or the heel of your hand. Use one hand as support on the back or shoulder area and work down one side at a time. Alternatively palm both sides at once, as shown on page 61.

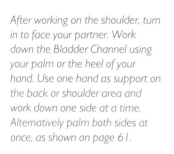

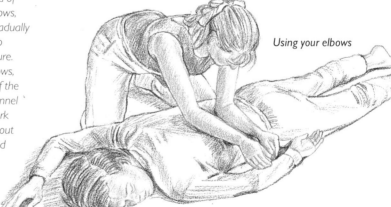

Palming the Bladder Channel

Some people with very tense or muscular backs may benefit from elbow pressure instead of thumbing. Position your elbows, relax your forearms, and gradually bring your weight forward to create perpendicular pressure. Ease back to shift your elbows, moving one a little ahead of the other as you follow the Channel down the back. You can work both sides of the spine without changing position. Relax and take your time.

Using your elbows

Thumbing the sacral points

Use both thumbs together to give pressure to the sacral points. They lie in two rows, one each side of the sacrum, in line with the main inner pathway of the Bladder Channel, and the other even closer

to the mid line (see p. 110).
    Shiatsu on the sacrum can help lower back pain, menstrual pain, and problems of the bladder and sexual organs.

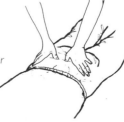

THE ASSOCIATED POINTS

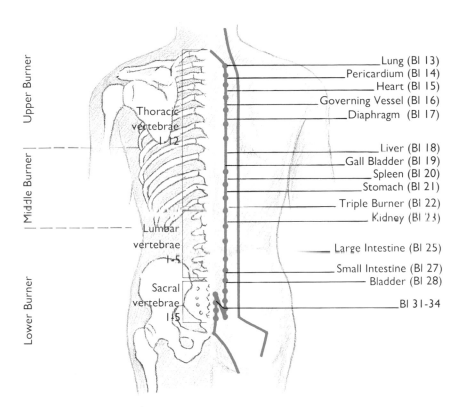

Upper Burner

Middle Burner

Lower Burner

Thoracic vertebrae 1-12

Lumbar vertebrae 1-5

Sacral vertebrae 1-5

Lung (Bl 13)
Pericardium (Bl 14)
Heart (Bl 15)
Governing Vessel (Bl 16)
Diaphragm (Bl 17)

Liver (Bl 18)
Gall Bladder (Bl 19)
Spleen (Bl 20)
Stomach (Bl 21)
Triple Burner (Bl 22)
Kidney (Bl 23)

Large Intestine (Bl 25)

Small Intestine (Bl 27)
Bladder (Bl 28)

Bl 31-34

The Bladder "associated points"

Twelve classically established points along the Bladder Channel relate directly to the twelve inner Organs. They are found along the inner line of the Bladder Channel down the back in three regions that correspond to the regions of the Triple Burner (see p. 132).

In the upper region, between the shoulder blades, level with the bony process of the 3rd, 4th, and 5th thoracic vertebrae, are points for the Lungs, Pericardium, and Heart. These are the Organs of the chest influencing circulation of Ki and Blood. The next two points also help circulation, especially Bl 17 (the Diaphragm Associated Point),

a very dynamic, strengthening, and regulating point for Blood.

In the middle region, level with the 9th to 12th thoracic vertebrae, are four associated points — for the Liver, Gall Bladder, Spleen, and Stomach. These work on the digestion, absorption, and distribution of nutrients.

The lower region is concerned with storage of reserves, sexual functions, drainage, and elimination. It is dominated by the Kidneys, with points level with the 2nd lumbar vertebra at the narrowest part of the waist, just above the hips. Just above are the points for the Triple Burner; these help regulate fluids. Those

of the Large Intestine, Small Intestine, Bladder, anus, and sacral region are found further down.

All these points carry Ki directly to the Organs, so they are sometimes called "Transporting Points". They can also be used for diagnosis. If an Organ is out of balance its associated point can become tender or sensitive to pressure. These points will help you develop an insight into your partner's general condition and so give effective treatments.

Work on the legs

To finish this routine, work down the Bladder and Kidney Channels on each leg. You can do this most effectively by treating first the Bladder Channel on the nearside and then, from the same position, leaning over to work down the Kidney Channel on the inner aspect of the opposite leg. Keep your supporting hand in touch with the sacral or lower lumbar region. Remember to change sides and work both Channels on both legs.

Preparation

Check that your partner's ankles are relaxed so the feet contact the floor when you lean on their legs. If not, provide support with a small cushion or rolled towel.

Lean with the palm or heel of the hand over the mid line of the thigh. Begin under the buttocks (see p. 64) and work toward the knee, calf, and ankle. Keep a wide base and avoid over-reaching.

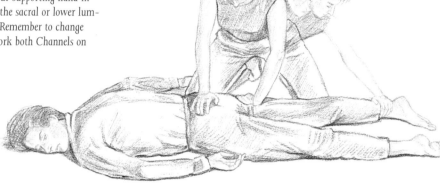

Palming the Bladder Channel

Thumbing the Bladder Channel

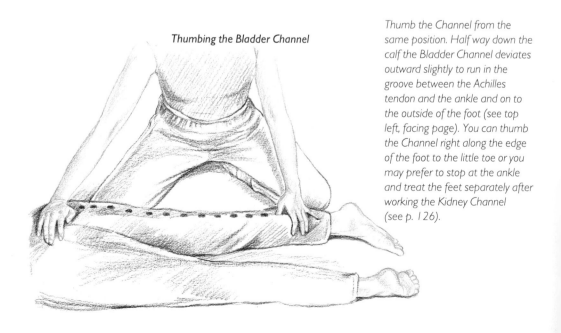

Thumb the Channel from the same position. Half way down the calf the Bladder Channel deviates outward slightly to run in the groove between the Achilles tendon and the ankle and on to the outside of the foot (see top left, facing page). You can thumb the Channel right along the edge of the foot to the little toe or you may prefer to stop at the ankle and treat the feet separately after working the Kidney Channel (see p. 126).

The Bladder Channel on the foot

The last section of the Bladder Channel influences the distant parts where the Channel begins.

Bl 60 ("Kun Lun Mountain") in the hollow between the ankle and the Achilles tendon strengthens the whole spine from sacrum to neck and helps ease a stiff neck and posterior headaches. It also helps to relieve menstrual pain, labour pains, and burning urination.

Bl 62 ("Extended Channel"), 1 in (2 cm) below the ankle tip, brings benefits to the whole back and relaxes the leg muscles. It also calms the mind and clears the eyes, helping reduce restlessness and insomnia if stimulated strongly (see also K 6, p. 127).

The remaining points, in the hollows between the muscle and bones along the edge of the foot, relieve congestion in the head, relax the neck, and calm the mind. They also clear the eyes when they are inflamed or blurry from the effects of wind, pollen, or acute infection.

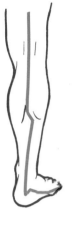

The Bladder Channel
in the leg

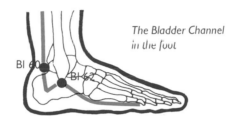

The Bladder Channel
in the foot

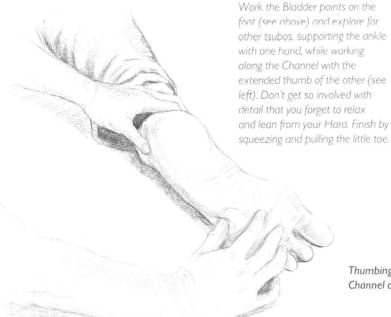

Work the Bladder points on the foot (see above) and explore for other tsubos, supporting the ankle with one hand, while working along the Channel with the extended thumb of the other (see left). Don't get so involved with detail that you forget to relax and lean from your Hara. Finish by squeezing and pulling the little toe.

Thumbing the Bladder
Channel on the foot

Treating the Kidneys

In addition to the common symptoms of Kidney deficiency (see p. 111) further symptom patterns characterize a weakness of either Yin or Yang Kidney functions.

Kidney Yang weakness manifests in fatigue, weak legs, cold feelings, frequent profuse urination or incontinence, low libido, or in men, a tendency to impotence.

Weak Kidney Yin produces dryness and thirst, night sweats, insomnia, chronic sore throats, flushed cheeks, scanty menstruation in women, and premature ejaculation in men.

It is important to treat the Bladder Channel in all Kidney problems, especially weakness of Yang. Kidney Yin deficiencies respond well to work on the leg, especially the Kidney points near the ankle. Rest and special exercises, such as Tai Chi, Chi Kung, or yoga are traditionally recommended for Kidney depletion.

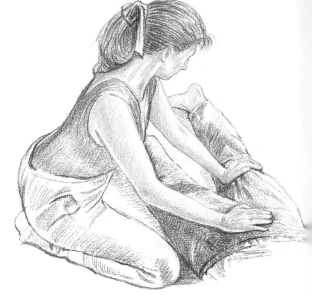

Palming the Kidney Channel

After palming and thumbing the Bladder Channel on the near leg, lean across to the opposite leg, to work on the Kidney Channel. Keep your support hand on the sacrum and palm down the inner aspect of the back of the thigh and leg.

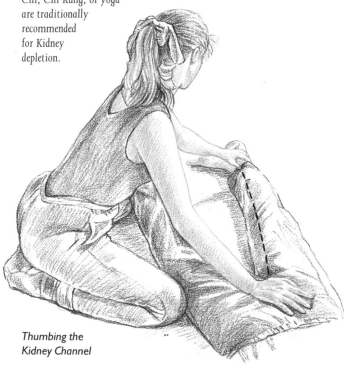

Thumbing the Kidney Channel

To "tonify" the Channel, relax, and work down slowly with the thumb. Feel for the deepest or most open tsubos and take time to let your pressure penetrate. Hold each one for several breaths. K 3 is the last point on the leg, behind the inner ankle (see left).

Repeat your work on the leg Channels on the other side. Then move on to the Bladder Channel (p. 125) and the Kidney Channel (facing page) on the foot.

Treating Kidney Yin deficiency

When in harmony, Yang is above and should go downward, Yin is below and moves upward, as in the normal direction of the Channels. Deficiency of Yin often causes the Yang Ki of the body to rise or rebel upward, causing unpleasant dry or hot symptoms in the head and disturbing the mind.

Typical patterns of Kidney Yin deficiency include chronic sore throat, thirst, flushed cheeks, and dry, sore eyes, restlessness, and insomnia. All the Kidney points around the inner ankle and on the foot tend to strengthen Yin and rectify this imbalance.

Kidney 1

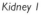

Kidney 1

This is another point that calms Yang and tonifies or strengthens the Yin. It is useful for someone in a particularly manic or disturbed state of restlessness, but it can also be

Kidney 6

Located in the hollow about 1 in (2 cm) below the tip of the inner ankle, this point sends Yin influence upward. It moistens the throat and eyes, calms the mind, and promotes sleep. If the person is particularly restless and tense, work more strongly first on the Bladder Channel, particularly Bl 62 (see p. 125).

Kidney 6 "Shining Sea"

helpful in shock or fainting, with headaches or nosebleeds, or exhaustion from heat.

K 1 is in the middle of the front part of the sole at the convergence of the lines made when the foot is flexed. Thumb systematically over the whole of the sole for a strengthening and calming influence (see also pp. 172–3).

This is a pleasant and effective alternative method if your thumbs are tired, or just for a change. Clasp under your partner's ankle with one hand as shown, keeping your hand on the floor for support. Then knead the whole underside of your partner's foot with the folded finger knuckles of the other hand, using your weight to apply a firm pressure.

Using the knuckles

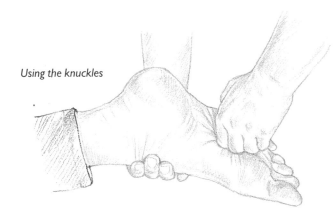

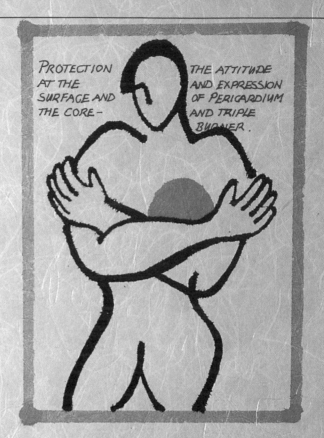

PROTECTION AT THE SURFACE AND THE CORE —

THE ATTITUDE AND EXPRESSION OF PERICARDIUM AND TRIPLE BURNER.

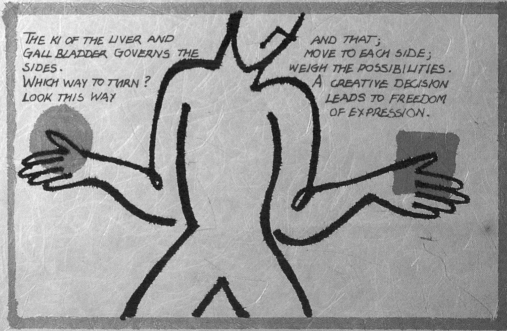

THE KI OF THE LIVER AND GALL BLADDER GOVERNS THE SIDES. WHICH WAY TO TURN? LOOK THIS WAY

AND THAT; MOVE TO EACH SIDE; WEIGH THE POSSIBILITIES. A CREATIVE DECISION LEADS TO FREEDOM OF EXPRESSION.

CHAPTER EIGHT

The Side Channels

PERICARDIUM · TRIPLE BURNER
GALL BLADDER · LIVER

The Channels of these four Organs form the last part of the cycle of Ki (see p. 79), flowing on the sides of the body between all the other Channels. The Pericardium and Triple Burner assist and protect. The Pericardium works for the Heart; it is the "Heart's Protector" from environmental heat, fevers, and emotional excesses. It mediates in social interaction like a minister to the monarch. The Triple Burner helps the Kidneys and protects the outside. It has no precise form, but harmonizes the functions of the body's upper, middle, and lower regions (see pp. 132-3). Its Ki assists transformation and regulates fluids in each region, co-operating with the Lungs, Spleen, and Kidneys. It is also an avenue for Kidney Ki to replenish the other Channels, warming and protecting the body surface.

The Pericardium and the Triple Burner both belong to the Fire element. Their "Minister" Fire is associated with Kidney Yang, the "Life-Gate Fire" of Mei Mon, and the Hara.

The Liver and Gall Bladder belong to the Wood element. Materially they store and distribute pure substances. The Liver stores Blood, releasing it to the muscles for activity. The Gall Bladder stores bile, which it releases for digestion.

Organs of creative action, skilful planning, wise judgement, and appropriate decisions, the Liver and Gall Bladder encompass destiny. Courageous decisions are the gift of the Gall Bladder. The Liver enables Ki to flow freely so that all body functions are smooth, and by its influence on planning, foresight and adaptability, makes an easy path through life.

The pathways for these four Channels are illustrated on pages 130–1 and 136–7; the Channel exercises are on pages 134–5 and 138–9. The routine begins on page 140.

The Pericardium Channel pathway

This Channel begins in the middle of the chest at the Pericardium. A branch descends internally through the diaphragm to the Upper, Middle, and Lower "Burners" — the three regions of the Triple Burner (see p. 132).

From the starting point a branch of the main Channel crosses the chest to emerge just outside the nipple. It then ascends on the surface around the front of the armpit and flows down the arm, through the biceps muscle. At the elbow crease it passes just to the inside of the biceps tendon (the Lung Channel is on the other side), then down the middle of the front of the forearm, between the Heart and Lung Channels (see pp. 106 and 84), to the wrist.

It crosses the middle of the palm to P 8 where it divides. The main Channel continues to the outer corner of the middle fingernail, and a connecting branch goes to the fourth finger to join the Triple Burner Channel at TB 1.

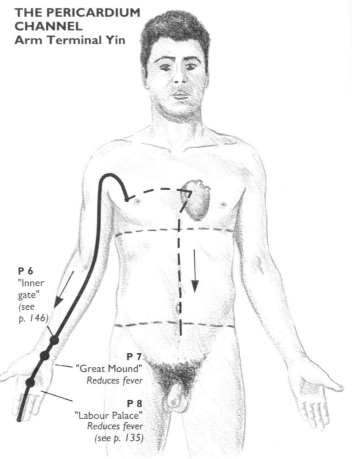

THE PERICARDIUM CHANNEL
Arm Terminal Yin

P 6
"Inner gate"
(see p. 146)

P 7
"Great Mound"
Reduces fever

P 8
"Labour Palace"
Reduces fever
(see p. 135)

The Pericardium Channel — functions and associated symptoms

The Pericardium is described as the Heart's "ambassador", bringing joy and happiness, helping to communicate our feelings, and protecting the Heart from emotional pain when relationships become stressful. To achieve this, the Pericardium Channel calms the Mind and balances the emotions, especially when there are relationship problems and break-ups (heartaches and heartbreaks).

As the Heart belongs to the Fire element it is vulnerable to extra Heat. The Pericardium's role as "Heart Protector" extends to absorbing Heat, to protect the Heart from attacks of fever. Most of the points along this Channel reduce hot symptoms associated with Heart or Blood disorders, and its last three points are specifically used for high fevers with great thirst, delerium, hallucinations, and restlessness, or prostration (e.g. sunstroke).

The Pericardium Channel has a wide influence on the chest. It eases chest tightness, stuffiness, or pains, whether caused by emotional stress, indigestion (heartburn), or phlegm.

The changing view of the Pericardium

The early classics constantly referred to the five Yin and the six Yang Organs. The Pericardium was seen as the Heart's protector and assistant, not an Organ in its own right. Some points on its Channel were originally ascribed to the Heart. However, the theory of the twelve Channels eventually demanded a symmetry that led to the pairing of the Pericardium with the Triple Burner Channel. Their relationship is not close, however, and their categorization under the Fire element (see p. 25) is for different reasons.

THE TRIPLE BURNER CHANNEL
Arm Lesser Yang

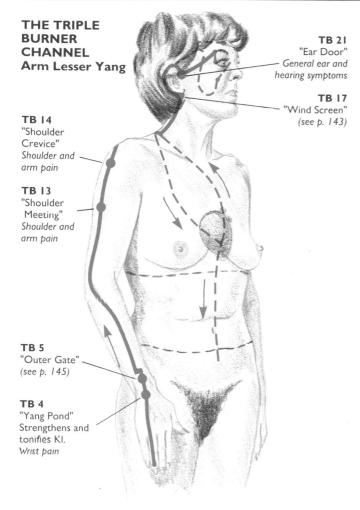

TB 21
"Ear Door"
General ear and hearing symptoms

TB 17
"Wind Screen"
(see p. 143)

TB 14
"Shoulder Crevice"
Shoulder and arm pain

TB 13
"Shoulder Meeting"
Shoulder and arm pain

TB 5
"Outer Gate"
(see p. 145)

TB 4
"Yang Pond"
Strengthens and tonifies KI.
Wrist pain

The Triple Burner Channel pathway

Beginning on the fourth finger, by the outside corner of the nail, the Triple Burner Channel passes between the knuckles of the fourth and fifth fingers to the wrist. From here it ascends between the two bones of the forearm (radius and ulna), through the tip of the elbow, and up the back of the arm to the shoulder. Behind the top of the shoulder it joins the Small Intestine and the Governing Vessel Channels. Then it rises over the shoulder to the collarbone region, descends internally to the Pericardium in the Upper Burner, and then to the abdomen and the Middle and Lower Burners (see p. 133).

Re-emerging from the chest at the collarbone, the Channel ascends the side of the neck and round the back of the ear. One branch rises internally to meet the Gall Bladder Channel on the forehead, then descends to join the Small Intestine Channel on the cheek. The superficial branch continues to the front of the ear and crosses to the outer corner of the eyebrow, where it joins the Gall Bladder Channel again, next in the cycle of energy flow (see p. 79).

The Triple Burner Channel – functions and associated symptoms

Symptoms of the Yang Channels often relate to their superficial pathways, and are connected with their role in defending the body from acute disease and environmental influences. The Triple Burner is no exception. Symptoms of this Channel include sore, red eyes, acute ear troubles or pain behind the ear, sore or swollen throat, and pains in the shoulder or arm, also symptoms of

chills and fevers, either acute or chronically recurring, sometimes with spontaneous sweating.

The Triple Burner transforms and regulates body fluids. It also assists the Kidneys, so treating it can move the Ki in the body's interior, especially the lower region. It can help when there is abdominal swelling and discomfort, sometimes with urination difficulties or constipation.

It also helps in weakness that is combined with an inability to stabilize body temperature and a susceptibility to infections and fevers. However, it is usually more effective to treat imbalances of the Three Burners by treating the Channels of the relevant Organs in each region.

The Triple Burner controversy

The Triple Burner has been the subject of much discussion and controversy in Chinese medicine. Some early classics described it as an Organ like other Yang Organs, with particular involvement in absorbing, metabolizing, and excreting fluids, but with no specific location (see below, left hand column). Others maintained that it was a generalization of the structure and energies of the upper, middle, and lower parts of the body — the "three regions" or "burners" — which included the functions of the Organs within each region (see below, right hand column).

Yet another classic (see quote, below) described it as an Organ with "a name but no form" and developed a more integrated view of the Triple Burner as an "avenue of Ki", assisting in all transformations by conducting basic, constitutional Ki from Mei-Mon, the "Life-Gate" in the Hara (see p. 53), to the other Organs. It helps extract Ki from air and food and assists in managing the body fluids and excreting waste, supporting the Lungs, Spleen, and Kidneys in the Upper, Middle, and Lower Burners respectively. Similarly, the Triple Burner conveys stored constitutional Ki to the twelve Channels when they are depleted, supplying energy for the body's defence in times of illness or stress.

THE "FLUID-REGULATING" MODEL OF THE TRIPLE BURNER

The Upper Burner is compared to a mist, as the Lungs disperse fluids to moisten the whole body, especially the skin.

The Middle Burner is compared to a muddy pool, steaming and bubbling like the activity of the Stomach and Spleen in digesting and separating food and fluids.

The Lower Burner is described as a drainage ditch, separating clean from dirty fluids and carrying away the waste.

THE "THREE BODILY REGIONS" MODEL OF THE TRIPLE BURNER

The upper region includes the chest, neck, and head, and the functions of the Lungs, Heart, and Pericardium. It "receives but does not expel".

The middle region comprises the area between the diaphragm and the navel and includes the functions of the Liver, Gall Bladder, Stomach, and Spleen. It "moves and transforms".

The lower region starts below the navel and includes the functions of the Large and Small Intestines, Bladder, and Kidneys. This region "excretes but does not receive".

The Tanden

"The Triple Burner is the avenue of food and drink, the beginning and the end of Ki"
CLASSIC OF DIFFICULTIES   c 100AD.

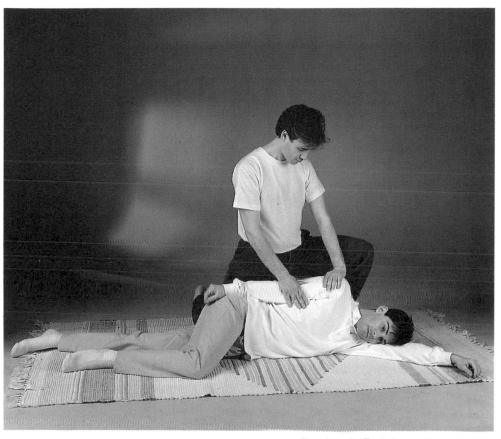

Thumbing the Triple Burner Channel

The Classic of Difficulties describes the Hara centre, or Tanden as the front focus of the "moving Ki between the Kidneys". According to the "avenue of Ki" model of the Triple Burner, this activates transformations in the three "burners" and nourishes all the Organs and their Channels, as shown symbolically by the arrow (see illustration left).

The role of the Liver
Some interpretations of the "bodily regions" model of the Triple Burner describe the Liver as part of the Lower Burner because of its strong influence on moving Ki and Blood in this area. The Liver has as much effect on the reproductive organs as do the Kidneys. Physically, however, it is in the middle region.

Understanding the Triple Burner
Consider the Triple Burner as a framework for understanding human physiology in the traditional Chinese way. Remember to think of both the general and the specific roles of all the Organs, and to see their overlapping and interacting functions as part of a harmonious system. Understanding this synthesis can help you interpret symptoms and therefore treat people more effectively.

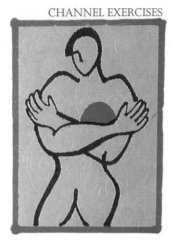

CHANNEL EXERCISES

Pericardium and Triple Burner

The first exercise on this page is a Makko Ho stretch to stretch and stimulate the Pericardium and Triple Burner Channels. Adapted from the posture of protection (see left), it symbolizes emotional defensiveness, dejection, or shyness and signifies huddling for warmth and protection from the elements.

The exercises that follow enhance our positive capacity to generate warmth and protection by building Ki through breathing, relaxed movement, and mental focus. The last in the sequence encourages an easy, rhythmic movement that loosens obstructed Ki, and lifts the spirit. The Pericardium influences circulation of Ki in the chest, the Triple Burner in the ribs and lower abdomen, and the Gall Bladder along the sides of the body and in the joints generally. This assists the Liver, which governs the smooth flow of Ki in the body.

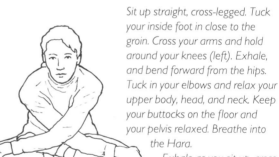

Sit up straight, cross-legged. Tuck your inside foot in close to the groin. Cross your arms and hold around your knees (left). Exhale, and bend forward from the hips. Tuck in your elbows and relax your upper body, head, and neck. Keep your buttocks on the floor and your pelvis relaxed. Breathe into the Hara.

Exhale as you sit up, cross your arms and legs the other way, and repeat.

Makko Ho

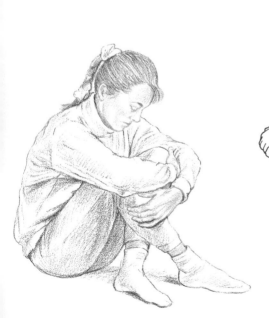

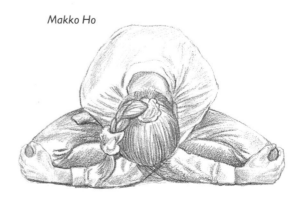

The Makko Ho stretch (see right) develops from the expression of the Pericardium and Triple Burner Channels (see above).

Pericardium 8, "Labour Palace", in the middle of the palms is regarded as an important focus for Ki. Rub your hands together in a relaxed but intent and purposeful way, keeping your breathing easy and deep. This soon produces warmth in the hands, increases their healing potential, and encourages Ki to circulate through your whole body.

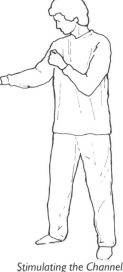

Form a loosely clenched fist and, keeping your wrist relaxed, beat your chest firmly from the centre of your breastbone (sternum) up and across to the front of your shoulder, then down the Pericardium Channel on the front of your arm to your palm. Turn your arm to beat its outer surface – the Triple Burner Channel – from wrist up to the shoulders. Finish by lifting your arm and beating down the Gall Bladder Channel on the side of the ribs.

*Stimulating the Channels
by beating*

Rubbing hands

Stand with your feet wide apart and parallel. Sink down a little, then relax your pelvis, and tuck your tailbone in. Turn your knees out slightly.

Now turn from the waist first to one side then the other. Let your arms swing naturally. Increase the movement, and eventually your arms will swing right round and slap your waist on the opposite sides.

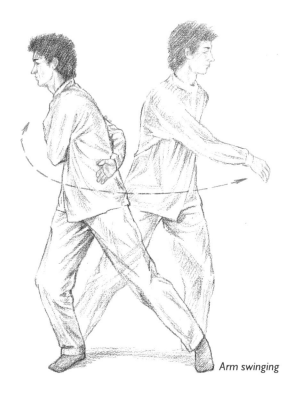

Arm swinging

The Gall Bladder Channel

This Channel begins just outside the outer corner of the eye, loops down and up to the forehead just within the hairline, and descends behind the ear to the corner of the skull. It then returns to the forehead above the centre of the eye and contours the head to the bottom of the skull at GB 20. It continues down the neck behind the shoulder to connect with the Governing Vessel at GV 14, then crosses over the shoulder. The Channel descends the side of the body along the rib margin to the waist and pelvic crest before going deeper to meet the Bladder Channel at the sacrum. At GB 30 it re-emerges and continues down the outside of the leg, in front of the ankle, ending on the outside of the 4th toe. Internal branches connect with the Stomach Channel (on the jaw) and the Small Intestine Channel, and join the Liver and Gall Bladder Organs.

Gall Bladder Channel – functions and associated symptoms

The Gall Bladder stores and secretes bile, which aids digestion, especially of fats. People with poor Gall Bladder function have difficulty digesting rich, fatty foods. This coincides with the Western medical view. Stagnation of Ki or Heat in the Gall Bladder can produce pain under the ribs, nausea and vomiting, a bitter or sour taste in the mouth, and yellow colour in the eyes.

The Gall Bladder influences the sides of the body and blockages or imbalances of the Gall Bladder Channel manifest in temple headaches, eye and ear pain, stiffness or pain in the jaw, shoulders, ribs, hips, or knee and ankle joints.

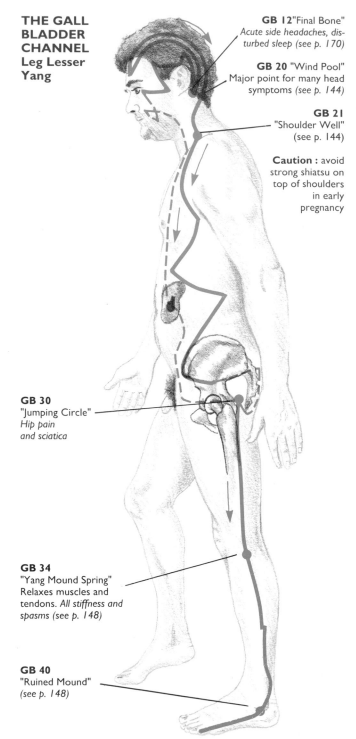

**THE GALL BLADDER CHANNEL
Leg Lesser Yang**

GB 12 "Final Bone"
Acute side headaches, disturbed sleep (see p. 170)

GB 20 "Wind Pool"
Major point for many head symptoms *(see p. 144)*

GB 21
"Shoulder Well"
(see p. 144)

Caution : avoid strong shiatsu on top of shoulders in early pregnancy

GB 30
"Jumping Circle"
Hip pain and sciatica

GB 34
"Yang Mound Spring"
Relaxes muscles and tendons. *All stiffness and spasms (see p. 148)*

GB 40
"Ruined Mound"
(see p. 148)

THE LIVER CHANNEL
Leg Terminal Yin

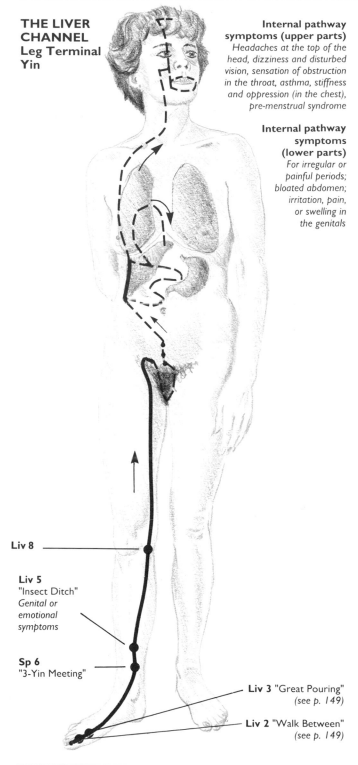

Internal pathway symptoms (upper parts)
Headaches at the top of the head, dizziness and disturbed vision, sensation of obstruction in the throat, asthma, stiffness and oppression (in the chest), pre-menstrual syndrome

Internal pathway symptoms (lower parts)
For irregular or painful periods; bloated abdomen; irritation, pain, or swelling in the genitals

Liv 8

Liv 5
"Insect Ditch"
Genital or emotional symptoms

Sp 6
"3-Yin Meeting"

Liv 3 "Great Pouring"
(see p. 149)

Liv 2 "Walk Between"
(see p. 149)

The Liver Channel pathway

Beginning by the inside of the big toenail the Liver Channel crosses the top of the foot, passes in front of the inside ankle and up the inner aspect of the leg through Sp 6 close behind the edge of the bone. It continues past the knee along the inner thigh to the groin and pubic region, where it circulates the external genitals. It connects with the Directing Vessel in the lower abdomen and continues up around the Stomach to enter both the Liver and Gall Bladder. Connecting with two surface points on the ribs, the Channel then dips into the ribcage, runs up through the throat, opening to the eye, and ends at the crown of the head where it connects with the Governing Vessel. A branch circles the mouth.

From within the Liver, another internal branch reaches the Lungs, and this restarts the cycle of Ki (see p. 79).

The functions of the Liver

The two principal functions of the Liver are storing Blood and helping all body functions run smoothly by spreading the Ki. The Liver also controls tendons and ligaments, and releases Blood to nourish these during activity, so that the joints and muscles work smoothly. Liver Blood also nourishes the eyes, to which the Liver "opens". The Blood returns to the Liver during rest.

Blockage of Ki causes Liver-related problems — aches, pains, and irregularity — in many parts of the body. The wide-ranging influence of Liver Ki can be seen by studying the course of its Channel.

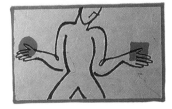

CHANNEL EXERCISES

Gall Bladder and Liver

The Liver guides our destiny; its role is associated with organization and planning. Its influence on the eyes not only relates to good sight but symbolically to insight and foresight. In this it is assisted by the Gall Bladder, with its influence over good judgement and decision making. The Liver has the overview while the Gall Bladder looks after the details.

Frustrations and difficulties can lead to anger, the powerful Liver emotion. Expressed appropriately, this can overcome obstacles and lead to creative solutions. However, unresolved difficulties block Liver Ki, and this results in depression. Irritability and unwarranted aggression come when the naturally expansive Wood energies find no proper outlet and rebel upward, often producing physical symptoms such as headaches.

Cowardice, timidity, and becoming "bogged-down" in details indicate weakness of the Gall Bladder.

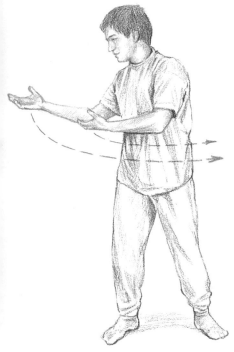

Relaxed stretches and exercises in easy coordinated movement benefit the Liver and Gall Bladder generally. Gentle "swing turns" (see above) open the sides and move the Ki. This exercise resembles the symbolic gesture – weighing up the alternatives, considering all the options.

Sit up with your legs stretched wide. Turn at the waist to face your left foot. Brace your left hand on the floor behind to lift your trunk and spine. Now wrap your right arm around your chest and ribs and inhale as you raise your left arm. Exhale slowly and lower your trunk and left arm in line with your right leg. Rest your arm over your head and relax for 2 or 3 breaths. Come out of the position and repeat on the other side.

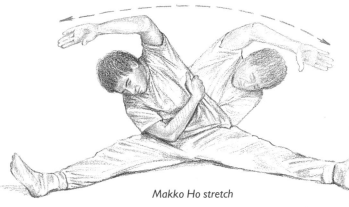

Makko Ho stretch

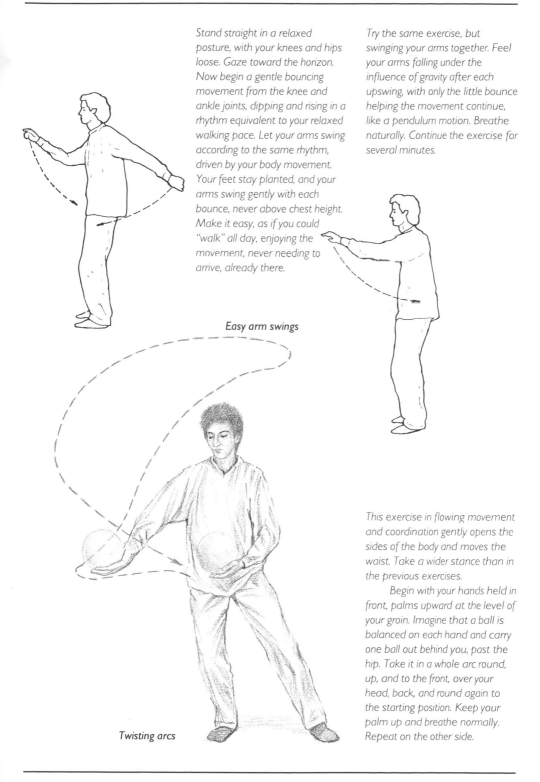

Stand straight in a relaxed posture, with your knees and hips loose. Gaze toward the horizon. Now begin a gentle bouncing movement from the knee and ankle joints, dipping and rising in a rhythm equivalent to your relaxed walking pace. Let your arms swing according to the same rhythm, driven by your body movement. Your feet stay planted, and your arms swing gently with each bounce, never above chest height. Make it easy, as if you could "walk" all day, enjoying the movement, never needing to arrive, already there.

Try the same exercise, but swinging your arms together. Feel your arms falling under the influence of gravity after each upswing, with only the little bounce helping the movement continue, like a pendulum motion. Breathe naturally. Continue the exercise for several minutes.

Easy arm swings

Twisting arcs

This exercise in flowing movement and coordination gently opens the sides of the body and moves the waist. Take a wider stance than in the previous exercises.

Begin with your hands held in front, palms upward at the level of your groin. Imagine that a ball is balanced on each hand and carry one ball out behind you, past the hip. Take it in a whole arc round, up, and to the front, over your head, back, and round again to the starting position. Keep your palm up and breathe normally. Repeat on the other side.

Shiatsu routine for the side Channels

The side position is especially useful for elderly people, pregnant women, and people with certain kinds of back pain, breathing troubles, or indigestion. It is particularly good for treating the four Channels in this chapter.

The Triple Burner and Gall Bladder have a strong influence on the sides of the body. They are implicated in many one-sided complaints or injuries.

The Pericardium and Liver Channels share an involvement in emotional expression. For sensitive people the giver's position behind the receiver can feel supportive and non-confrontational, while permitting some deeply effective shiatsu.

Use a pillow to support your partner's head. Find the most stable position for your partner by bringing the lower shoulder forward slightly to rest on the ground, and folding the top leg forward in front of the outstretched lower leg.

Kneel close by your partner's back, resting your nearside hand on the shoulder and placing your other between the shoulder blades, the area corresponding with the Heart and Pericardium. Pause for a moment.

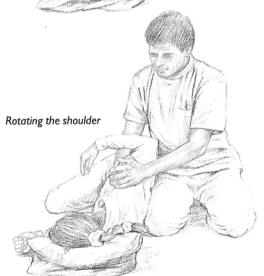

Rotating the shoulder

Insert your arm under your partner's armpit to support the front of the shoulder. Clasp the shoulder with both hands and begin to move it slowly in circles. Use your Hara and your body movement to follow and feel the limits of the motion and rotate the joint more widely – a few times in each direction.

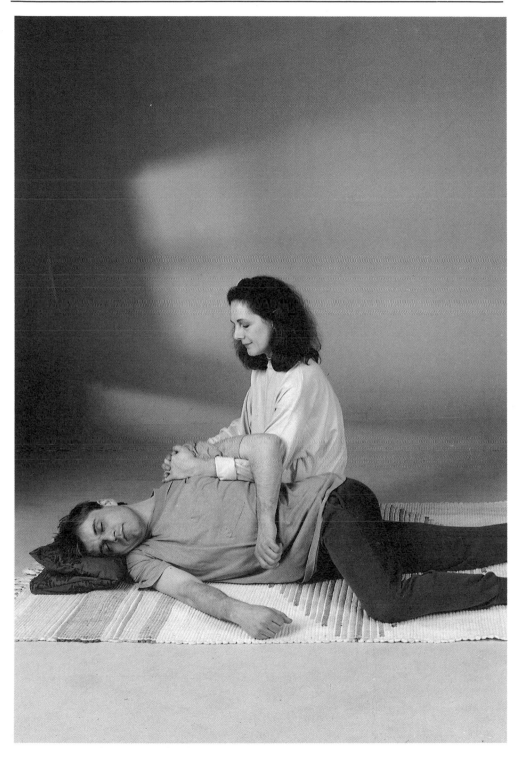

Rotating the shoulder in the side position.

Palming the side of the head opens both of the Yang Channels (Triple Burner and Gall Bladder) that cross it. Kneel up and step forward with your outer leg. Support your partner with the thigh of your other leg. Place your palms comfortably on your partner's head (see right). Lean and palm gently around the side of the head.

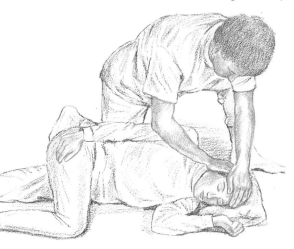

Palming the side of the head

Positioning the support hand

In this part of the routine your near-side hand always plays the supporting role. Tuck your elbow against your partner's shoulder and place your support hand behind the head while your active hand works on parts in front of the ear.

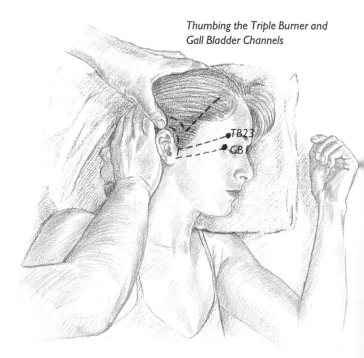

Thumbing the Triple Burner and Gall Bladder Channels

Begin at TB 23, the small hollow near the outer end of the eyebrow, and follow the path of the Triple Burner (see p. 131) down to the front of the ear then around to TB 17. Return to GB 1, level with the outer corner of the eye, and thumb this Channel down to the hollow in front of the ear, then up to the forehead and back around the ear. Work a little outside the TB Channel as shown, to GB 12 at the corner of the skull.

Shiatsu on the head

Even on the head there are subtle hollows and dents that correspond to the joints in the skull. Feel with sensitivity for these points as you go. Use relaxed leaning pressure into those you can feel. The skin and underlying membranes and muscles of the head are very lively and responsive. This makes work on the head very rewarding.

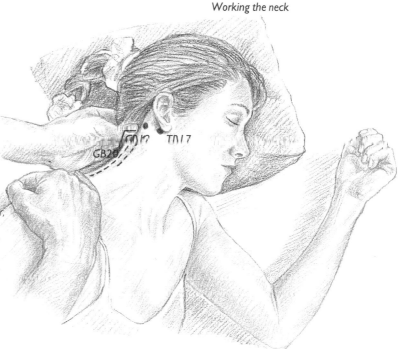

Working the neck

Sit back slightly and cup your support hand around the shoulder, then lean back a little to "open" the neck. With the fingers of your working hand you can give quite firm pressure to the tsubos under the base of the skull, particularly GB 12 and GB 20 (see right). Work down the neck, at first just resting your thumb across the sterno-cleido-mastoid muscle using the relaxed weight of your arm. Then, working a little more firmly with extended thumb, give pressure behind the muscle to the TB Channel (see p. 131).

Return to the base of the skull and follow the GB Channel (see p. 136), leaning with the thumb in a similar way into the groove between the neck muscles.

TB 17 ("Wind Screen")

Located in the hollow between the corners of the jawbone and skull, behind the ear lobe, this sensitive but important point is useful for all ear troubles including pain from exposure to wind — hence its name. Press gently but firmly with the tip of your thumb or forefinger.

GB20 ("Wind Pool")

Located under the skull in the large hollow between the muscles, this is one of the most important points for the head. With a strong clearing and dispersing action, it is helpful for all headaches, including migraine. Use it also for eye troubles, ear problems, or stuffiness, pain, or blockage of the nose and sinuses, acute or chronic.

Squat and turn to face your partner's feet. Rest your near hand over the head, curling your fingers under the base of the skull. With the thumb of the other hand work the TB and GB Channels across the top of the shoulder, inching along from the corner of the neck as far as the bony extremity.

Caution

GB 21, which is at the top of the shoulder, near the neck, should not be pressed during the early stages of pregnancy or whenever there is threatened miscarriage. It is useful, however, during labour as part of an "inducing" treatment.

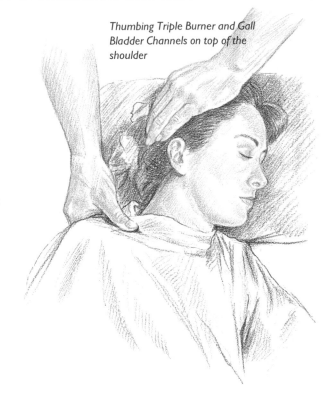

Thumbing Triple Burner and Gall Bladder Channels on top of the shoulder

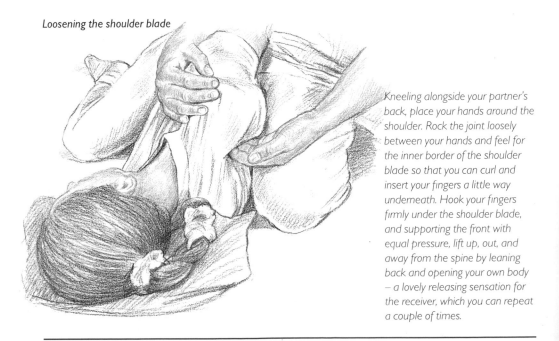

Loosening the shoulder blade

Kneeling alongside your partner's back, place your hands around the shoulder. Rock the joint loosely between your hands and feel for the inner border of the shoulder blade so that you can curl and insert your fingers a little way underneath. Hook your fingers firmly under the shoulder blade, and supporting the front with equal pressure, lift up, out, and away from the spine by leaning back and opening your own body – a lovely releasing sensation for the receiver, which you can repeat a couple of times.

The Triple Burner Channel

To treat this Channel, rest the arm along your partner's side, wrist over the hip. Kneel up behind, with your knees wide spaced, and steady your partner's shoulder with your supporting hand. The Channel runs just to the rear of the mid line of the shoulder muscle (deltoid), down to the bony point of the elbow.

Palm the outer arm from the shoulder muscle to the wrist. Then kneel back slightly to thumb the Channel in the upper arm. To follow the Channel from the elbow, kneel up close and lean directly down, thumbing along the space between the two bones of the forearm to the hollow at the wrist where the tendons of the hand converge.

Thumbing the Triple Burner Channel on the arm

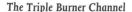

TB 5 ("Outer Gate")

The most versatile, wide acting point of the Triple Burner Channel is found 2 in (5 cm) above the wrist, between the bones (see above). Useful in acute, feverish conditions, with chills, sore throat, and sweating, and as a "distant point" for earache, side headaches, swollen glands, and stiff neck. It is also good for pain in the ribs, shoulder, or wrist.

Continue toward the space between the knuckles of the 4th and 5th fingers and finish by squeezing the sides of the 4th finger.

The Pericardium Channel

This Channel runs right through the mid line of the biceps muscle on the upper arm, passing to the inside of the tendon at the elbow. Then it runs along the middle inside aspect of the forearm, between the two prominent tendons above the wrist (P 6), across the middle of the palm, and along the middle finger.

Start work on this Channel by rotating the shoulder (see p. 120), finishing with your partner's arm across your lap.

At first palm the Channel with your thumb laid flat across the inner arm, exerting general pressure while your fingers support behind. Return to the top and thumb the Channel at a more penetrating angle. Keep your shoulder relaxed.

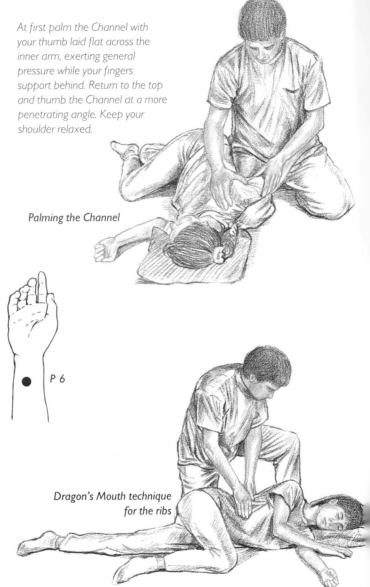

Palming the Channel

Pericardium 6 ("Inner Gate")

This point is situated approximately 2in (5cm) above the inner wrist crease, between the two prominent tendons of the lower arm.

It has a strong influence on the whole chest area, and "harmonizes the Stomach". Use this point when indigestion causes nausea, acidity, and heartburn. It is also valuable as first aid for morning sickness and travel sickness.

P 6 moves Ki and Blood and calms the Mind. It helps anxiety, depression, and all kinds of emotional problems, especially when accompanied by tightness, heaviness, or pain in the chest. It also relieves pre-menstrual syndrome with distention or pain in the breasts.

P 6

Dragon's Mouth technique for the ribs

This two-handed version of the "Dragon's Mouth" (see p. 46) is ideal for working the GB Channel on the sides and helps move Ki in the chest. After working down the arm, lift and rotate it once or twice more then place it down comfortably in front. Kneel up and lean with both hands spread over the side of the ribs (see above), as you work down from the armpit to the waist. Keep both hands together and give your partner time to breathe with the movement. Be firm yet relaxed – light pressure is ticklish.

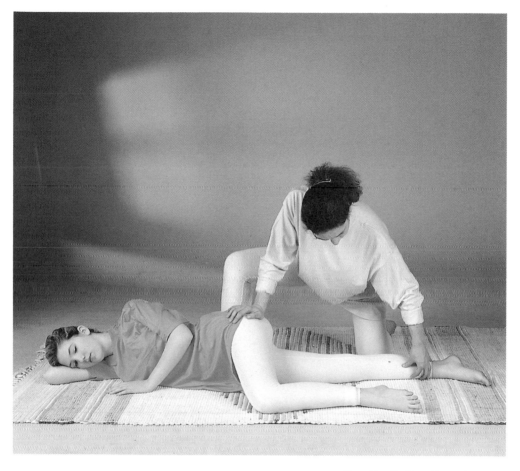

Thumbing the Liver Channel

Positioning for the
Gall Bladder Channel

While working down this Channel in the leg, your supporting hand can rest usefully on the classical point GB 30 situated on the outside of the buttock, just above and behind the prominent hip bone. It acts on all the leg joints and also benefits the lower back. It has a strengthening and comforting effect. Sciatic pain often follows the path of the Gall Bladder Channel. In this case, palming is the best general technique — use your thumbs sparingly if the pain is bad.

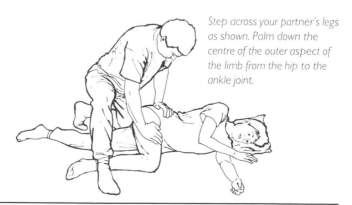

Step across your partner's legs as shown. Palm down the centre of the outer aspect of the limb from the hip to the ankle joint.

After palming, thumb the Channel down to the knee. Below the knee, locate GB 34 (see below). From here work down toward the ankle, along the bony edge of the fibula. Cross in front of the ankle and thumb down to the space between the 4th and 5th toes. Pull and squeeze the 4th toe. Always consider working the lower GB Channel for acute headaches, eye troubles, insomnia, and irritability.

Thumbing the Gall Bladder in the leg

GB 34 ("Yang Mound Spring")

On the outside of the leg, 2in (5cm) below the kneecap, GB 34 is found in the hollow immediately below and just in front of the head of the fibula, a small bony prominence – the "Yang Mound" of the point's name.

This point helps the Liver smooth the flow of Ki. It is generally relaxing and has a special action on all tendons and muscles. It helps in sprains and strains, pain and stiffness of any joints, muscular spasms, abdominal cramps, and constipation. It also benefits Gall Bladder symptoms such as biliousness and indigestion pains below the ribs.

GB 40 ("Ruined Mound")

Immediately below and to the front of the outer ankle bone, GB 40 strengthens the Gall Bladder and is useful for many problems occurring along the Channel. It is a good "distant point" for knee and hip pains, rib pains, stiff neck, and shoulders. It can also help people who lack the courage of their convictions and fail to make decisions, or become overwhelmed by details.

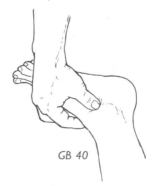

GB 40

The Liver Channel in the lower leg

Work on the Liver Channel affects all areas of the body as it promotes the free flow of Ki. Particular areas of benefit are the lower abdomen, including bowel and bladder function, but especially irregularity and pain of menstruation in women, also the external genitals of both sexes, the chest and ribs, the throat, eyes, and the top of the head. Troubles in any of these areas, especially if they are associated with frustration, depression, sudden outbursts of anger, or any other emotional stress, indicate involvement of the Liver. Stress blocks the Ki causing pain and irregularity.

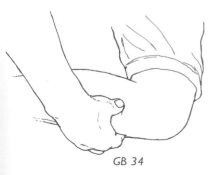

GB 34

Palm the Channel along the inside leg, leaning into the relaxed tendon of the upper thigh, down past the knee and on to the calf, then close behind the bone on the lower leg to the ankle. Keep your support hand on the sacral region.

Thumbing the Liver Channel

Thumb along the border of the tendon near the groin, along the middle of the inner thigh to the knee. Work into the classical point, Liver 8, in the end of the knee crease. The Channel runs on down the calf muscle behind the Spleen Channel, but about halfway down, it crosses in front of the Spleen Channel to continue very close behind the edge of the bone. Joining the Spleen Channel at Sp 6, "3-Yin Meeting", it then crosses in front of the ankle, over the top of the foot to the big toe.

Ask your partner to turn briefly to the supine position before moving to the other side to repeat the whole routine. At the end, work on both feet with your partner in the supine position (see below).

Thumbing the Liver Channel

Working on the feet

With your partner lying supine you can give special attention at the end of your session to the feet, which have particular significance for the Liver. Both the Liver and Gall Bladder can be upset by rich and spicy foods, stimulant drugs, and alcohol. These, along with the emotions, can combine to overheat the Liver. Its Yang energy then rises forcefully to the head causing acute headaches, sore eyes, dizziness, and nausea. This sounds like a hangover, and it could be, on occasions of excess. But more serious and chronic disharmonies can result in similar symptoms in the long term. Migraines are often a result of the over-stressed lifestyle of busy, creative people who work hard and play hard. Unpredictable moods, irritability, insomnia, red eyes, and indigestion are common symptoms of the Liver on overdrive – called "Liver Fire rising". The last few tsubos on the Liver and Gall Bladder Channels (see facing page) can reduce Liver Fire.

Liver 3 ("Great Pouring")

Working on this point increases the Yin of the Liver – Liver Blood. This nourishes tendons and ligaments, helping all tightness, tension, and spasms. It spreads Liver Ki, reducing pains and obstruction along its Channel and helps regularity and smoothness of all its functions. It eases emotional stress and helps all headaches whether due to excess or weakness.

Liver 2 ("Walk Between")

This is more useful when symptoms are acute, irritating, dry, or hot. It is the "Fire point" of the Liver Channel. Use it with Liver 3 for bad headaches, period pains, nausea, or painful, difficult urination.

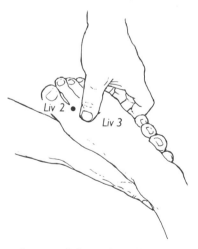

Rotate each foot at the ankle joint, then grasp and stretch each one in turn, first away from the body, leaning back, then toward the head. Press the Liver tsubos calmly and methodically. Hold the feet for a moment to finish.

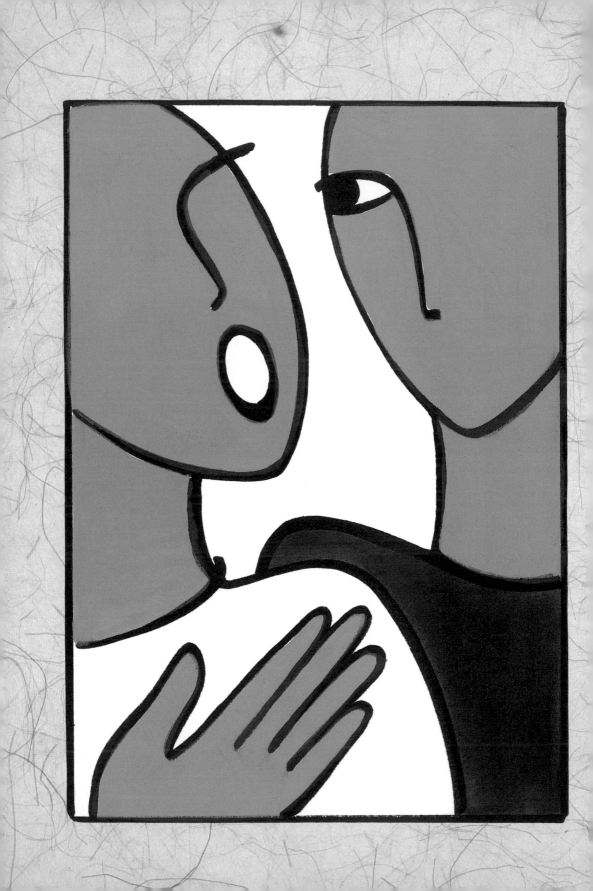

PART THREE

Versatility with Simplicity

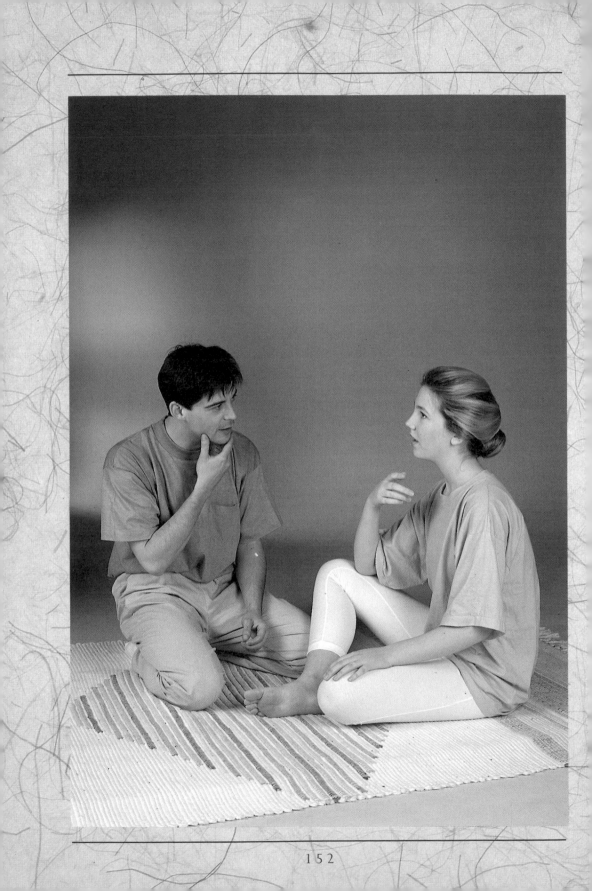

CHAPTER NINE

A Guide
to Diagnosis

One of the highest goals of Chinese medicine is to help others to live in harmony with the Tao, the Way of Nature. The illnesses that we all experience from time to time are part of this Way. We progress through a series of imbalances, larger or smaller, just as the weather, manifesting the changing seasons, is sometimes rough, violent, unpredictable, but still part of the overall harmony of nature. Our illnesses represent an opportunity to learn about ourselves, and to change and improve our lifestyles. In the West our attempts to banish sickness from our lives ignore the real possibilities for improvement that these illnesses bring.

We mistake the symptoms of an illness for the disease itself. Our medicinal drugs, an armoury of painkillers, anti-biotics, anti-inflammatories, anti-histamines, and anti-depressants, with all their attendant side-effects, suppress and confuse the body's clear expression that all is not well inside. Or we may ignore our troubles in the hope that they will go away. Whichever route we take, the constitution has limits: we can only go on like this for so long.

Traditional Chinese medicine relates the events in our bodies to our lives and the environment (see p. 17). It interprets symptoms and signs as a signature of underlying disharmony but accepts these changes as fundamental. Your shiatsu treatment helps to restore balance and harmony in your partner. The traditional causes of disease are described on pages 155–9. Diagnostic methods are discussed on pages 160–5.

For readers of this book it is important to use the information wisely. It is intended to provide guidelines for your work. Use it in the spirit of humility, as a way of understanding your shiatsu partner's immediate needs and as a basis for discussion of lifestyle and the possible causes of illness. If you are not a professional then advise friends to seek help from a skilled practitioner if necessary. Your shiatsu can still be of valuable help.

The traditional causes of disease

Understanding the causes of disease helps you interpret the particular symptoms and signs that the body produces as an indication of disharmony. By recognizing the origin of the disharmony, the sick person can make adjustments that will speed recovery and improve his or her health and resistance. This may involve alterations in diet, activities, or attitudes – habitual ways of being in, or relating to, the world. In this way, illness can be used as a catalyst for positive change.

The nine main causes of disease are divided into internal and external categories, plus miscellaneous causes (see below). Each upsets the functions of the Organs and Channels in specific ways (see pp. 155–9). Their effects are either more Yin or more Yang. Emotions, climate, and diet form part of the picture of connections with the Five Elements, as described and illustrated in this section. Refer back to page 24 for the progression of illnesses through the Five Element sequences.

Resistance
The severity of symptoms reflects the strength of the disease relative to the person's resistance, and the degree of struggle between them.

Weak people will be susceptible to milder adverse influences. Their symptoms will tend to be mild but more persistent. But if the Ki and Blood are strong, and the mind flourishing, a person will be more adaptable and able to withstand greater extremes.

However, excessive demands of work, emotional stress, poor diet, or climatic exposure may overwhelm or wear down even the strongest individuals. Their illnesses will tend to be more dramatic but short-lived, as they recover quickly.

INTERNAL CAUSES

The seven emotions
Joy, Overthinking, Worry, Sadness, Fear, Fright, Anger

Poor or inappropriate diet

Overwork

Excess sexual activity

Weak constitution

EXTERNAL CAUSES

The six climatic factors
Heat and Fire, Dryness, Wind, Cold, Damp

MISCELLANEOUS CAUSES

Poisoning; insect, snake, and animal bites

Trauma, injury

Wrong treatment

EXTERNAL CAUSES – THE CLIMATIC FACTORS

The weather is the Ki of the outer environment. Our bodies adapt naturally to the climate and normally we can use our common sense to dress according to the prevailing conditions. But sometimes even the mildest change in the weather may catch us unprepared and upset our equilibrium, especially if we are run down and our defences are low. The Yang Channels and the Lungs are the most important lines of defence.

The Yang Channels

Yang protects the outside; Yin nourishes the inside. The Yang Channels circulate the outer and upper parts of the body and play a role in defence generally. Climatic excesses usually affect the upper part of the body (except for Damp which often rises from the earth and affects the joints in the lower body). Therefore acute disease caused by the weather is often best treated by the Yang Channels.

The Lungs

External factors and acute illness do not usually affect the Yin Organs directly, but the Lungs are an exception. They are situated highest in the body like a protective "lid" and open to the exterior. They are the most Yang of the Yin Organs.

The Lungs circulate "Protective Ki", which fights the invading influence. Frequent coughs, colds, or fevers are a sign of weak Lungs and Protective Ki.

Internal correspondences

A Yin-Yang disharmony within the body, when associated with weak functioning of the Organs, may produce symptoms very similar to the external climates. Because of this, they are referred to as interior Damp, interior Wind, and so on. These conditions affect the Yin Organs as often as the Yang.

THE EFFECT OF CLIMATE ON BODY

Climatic excess	Symptoms and associations	Element	Channels & Organs affected
HEAT & FIRE	High temperature, fever, thirst, red face, and skin rashes, profuse sweating, fear of heat, irritability, restlessness. Extreme Heat invades the Pericardium causing delerium and collapse (as in sunstroke).	FIRE	Heart Small Intestine Triple Heater Pericardium
DRYNESS	Similar to Heat but milder. Prolonged Heat or fever – dry Large Intestine: dry skin, lips, and throat, constipation; dry Stomach: nausea and dry mouth; dry indoor heating or warm, dry wind – Lungs: dry cough.	METAL	Large Intestine Lungs
WIND	The most vicious climatic excess; its drives other influences in and unpredictable, sudden, and violent symptoms come and go, and move about. Headaches, stuffy or streaming nose, sneezing, stiff neck, dizziness, itching, spasms, tics, and fear of wind.	WOOD	Gall Bladder Liver
COLD	Fevers – the main symptoms are chills, shivering, little or no sweating, and fear of cold. Cold causes contraction and blocks the flow of Ki: cramps, spasms, and fixed pains in the joints. Cold affects the Water element: profuse, pale urination, pain, watery colds, and feeling chilled to the bone.	WATER	Bladder Kidneys
DAMP	Damp housing conditions, sitting or sleeping on damp ground, as well as prolonged damp weather produce symptoms that are sluggish in onset and are difficult and slow to cure. They often affect the lower body and limbs: swelling, numbness, feelings of heaviness, stiff, swollen joints, tiredness, and sometimes a dull, heavy headache. Internally Damp attacks the Spleen: phlegm, excessive mucus, and discharges.	EARTH	Stomach Spleen

The seven emotions

Your emotions enable you to communicate your deep feelings. If they are repressed, the emotions persist and may become unbalanced.

Oriental medicine associates the emotions with the Yin Organs at the core of your being. Each Organ is connected with a particular emotion (see the Five Element Chart, p. 25), but two Organs bear the brunt of all emotional difficulties – the Heart and Liver.

Treating the appropriate Organs along their Channels can support people through emotionally stressful times, helping to regulate imbalances, and prevent further upset. The close, supportive contact that shiatsu offers can be invaluable in times of stress.

Joy
This is the emotion of the Heart. It calms the Mind and relaxes the Ki. The Heart's "ambassador", the Pericardium, brings joy and happiness to the Heart by mediating and regulating relationships. Excessive stimulation of the senses or passionate over-indulgence in excitement and pleasure are said to distract and unsettle the Mind and disturb the Heart, causing its Fire to flare up. Over-exuberance suggests a Heart imbalance.

Sadness or grief
Sadness results from disappointment, or more seriously from separation and loss. It is said to "dissolve" the Ki and principally affects the Lungs, expressed in its "sound" – weeping (see p. 25). Sadness is felt in the Heart and affects the whole chest, producing heaviness, breathlessness, tiredness, and depression. We need time to express our sadness or grief; rituals for dealing with change and loss probably help us to cope better with these emotions.

Worry
Worry springs from insecurity and tends to deplete the Spleen, which belongs to the Earth element and which in turn relates to support, nourishment, and early nurture. Worry "knots" the Ki of the Lungs, tightening the chest and shoulders and constricting breathing. We can feel immobilized by worry. The Lungs and the Spleen are the sources of the body's True Ki, so worry depletes Ki generally.

Pensiveness
This emotion is similar to worry but relates specifically to our capacity for mental work. The Spleen governs the intellect and so can suffer from the effects of overthinking, made worse by lack of exercise and irregular meals. The results are weakness, indigestion, and phlegm.

A weak Spleen can manifest as obsession with order and detail – the making of endless lists, calorie counting, or computer hobbyists becoming "hooked to their screens".

Fear
Fear is associated with the Kidneys. It makes Ki descend and affects the "pit of the Stomach".

In children it can manifest as night fears and bed-wetting. Adults with Kidney deficiency and weak constitutions may also be prone to "irrational" fears and anxiety, insomnia, spontaneous sweating, and dry mouth.

Unacceptable fear is sometimes unconsciously transferred into a strong drive to undertake dangerous occupations or pastimes, which justify the confrontation of fear. But if the root of the fear is not recognized, Kidney Yang can deplete the Yin, causing "uprising Fire" problems in the Liver and Heart.

Fright
This emotion is similar to fear but more extreme. It is identical to shock, associated with physical or emotional trauma. It suspends or scatters the Ki and affects the Kidneys and the Heart. The Kidneys store Ki for defence and may be suddenly drained. The Heart suffers from disruption of the Mind.

Emotions of the Heart and Liver

The Heart is associated with love, warmth, and the formation of relationships. It houses the Mind, or Spirit, which governs general stability. Emotional stress and shock can lead to mental disturbance, anxiety, and unstable behaviour.

The Liver governs the free flow of Ki. Emotional stress and general frustrations restrain the Liver and block Ki. This can cause pain, stuffiness, or obstruction anywhere in the body, as well as depression or forceful explosions of feeling.

Shock is characterized by loss of memory, disorientation, palpitations, dizziness, trembling, sweating, and fainting. Unresolved shock ties up the energy, which causes depletion.

Anger

This is the emotion of the Liver. It can take several modified forms, including irritability, frustration, jealousy, and rage. Anger makes the Ki rise, and with it the bile. A bitter taste in the mouth, red or yellowish eyes, redness of the face and neck, dizziness, and especially headaches are symptoms and signs of "rebellious" Liver Ki.

If suppressed the Yang dynamic of anger turns into the Yin state of depression, which causes stagnation of Liver Ki and aches, pains, and feelings of oppression, stuffiness, or bloatedness. Either form of Liver emotion can upset the Stomach and Spleen. Its Wood energy expands and then "invades" the Earth Organs (see p. 24) causing nausea, acidity, vomiting, or diarrhoea.

CONSTITUTION

Life begins at conception. In the womb the fetus is nourished by "Prenatal Ki", the foundation of the constitution, stored in the Kidneys in the form of Essence. The parents' health, especially that of the mother during pregnancy, and the circumstances of birth establish initial constitutional strength and determine the amount of Prenatal Ki. This is supplemented after birth by Postnatal Ki from air and food. Serious illnesses or accidents may weaken constitutional Ki. It may also be squandered by careless living. However, careful diet and avoidance of extremes conserves it. Teachers of internal exercise systems such as Chi Kung or Tai Chi claim that these increase constitutional reserves.

A weak constitution renders a person more susceptible to illness and this weakness can be a specific cause of Kidney disease.

EXCESS SEX AND OVERWORK

The Kidneys are most affected by these two causes of disease, which can be considered together as they sometimes complicate each other.

Kidney Essence forms the sexual fluids and reproductive substances of both sexes. Kidney Yang provides the energy for sex. The Kidneys are associated with physical drive, including the ability to cope with energetic work. Hard physical work, lifting and bending, or jobs that involve standing for long periods can deplete them. Overdemanding mental work depletes the Spleen as well as the Kidneys.

"Excessive sex" requires common sense in its interpretation. It depends on age, constitutional strength, and circumstance. Traditionally, men deplete their Essence through ejaculation, but excessive orgasm weakens the Kidneys in both

sexes. Too many late nights, sex while drunk, or when tired from overwork can all be contributory factors.

Women lose less of their sexual fluids during sex and so tend to recover more quickly, but they can suffer from the physical demands of pregnancy, which also depletes the Essence. Childbirth, feeding, and caring for young children also make great demands.

MISCELLANEOUS CAUSES

These include bites and poisons, trauma, epidemics, and wrong treatment. Wrong treatment is as prevalent today as it has ever been. Illnesses that are caused by wrong treatment are known as iatrogenic diseases.

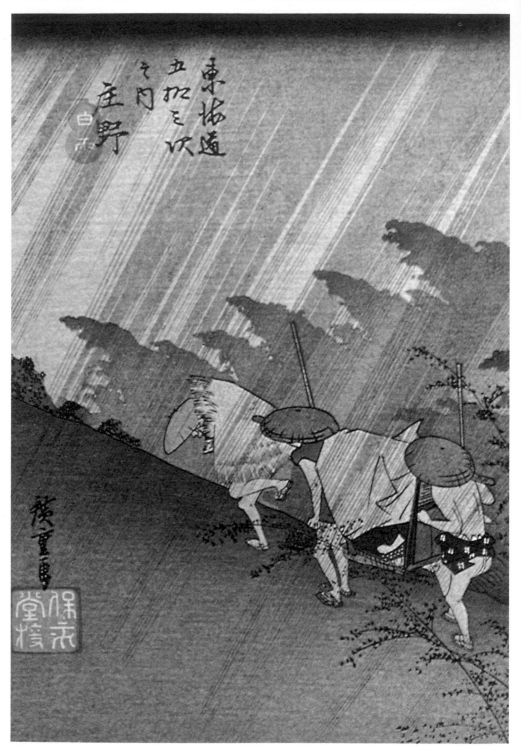

The impact of the weather is acknowledged in much Oriental art.

DIET

Our technological advances have led us down the path of consuming processed, de-natured, reconstructed, additive-laced foods that generally lower health and resistance to disease. The proliferation of dietary theories, books, special regimes, food substitutes, and supplements confuses most people, and produces a dependency on special products and "expert" advice.

In the face of this, traditional Chinese medicine offers a refreshingly down-to-earth approach to diet, advocating balance, moderation, and common sense.

The balance of Yin and Yang in food is shown in the chart (right). The foods in the central area of the chart are more balanced than those at the top and bottom. But even the extreme foods can be eaten and enjoyed in moderation.

Our diet can create problems if we eat mostly Yin or mostly Yang foods; so can habitually eating our meals too fast, or eating while angry, anxious, or under stress, late in the day, or at irregular times. Eat regularly, chew slowly and allow time for digestion. In this way all kinds of foods can be tolerated.

Five Element theory categorizes foods according to flavour, listing "five tastes" associated with the Five Elements (see chart below). A little of each flavour nourishes its associated Yin Organ but excesses unbalance the cycle, causing trouble in any related Organs. Cravings are manifestations of imbalance.

YIN AND YANG INFLUENCE IN FOODS

Rich, spicy and hot foods increase Yang in the body. They put stress on the Liver, aggravate "hot" illnesses and create phlegm.

red meats   greasy fried foods   black pepper
chilli pepper   garlic   cinnamon   coffee
red wine and spirits

Yang Extreme   baked and roasted foods

white wine and aperitifs

chicken   peaches   cooked whole grains, flakes

lamb   beef   grapes   rice   peas

corn   beans

root vegetables   oats   potatoes

dates, raisins   wheat

honey   millet   leafy vegetables

nuts and seeds   barley

celery   asparagus

milk   buckwheat

eggs   flours, bread, pasta   apples   fruit juices

white fish   pork   pears   mineral waters

boiled foods   raw foods   beers

herbal teas   **Yin Extreme**

ice cream   iced drinks   sugary drinks   colas

salt   seaweeds and shellfish   water

melon   banana   cucumber   tomato

lettuce   cold, raw foods

Cold, fresh, and raw foods put stress on the Spleen. Too many Yin foods aggravate "cold" conditions with poor circulation, weak digestion with loose bowels, and damp, watery, or phlegmy illnesses.

Five Element flavour associations

Element	Earth	Metal	Water	Wood	Fire
Organ	Spleen	Lung	Kidney	Liver	Heart
Flavour	Sweet	Pungent	Salt	Sour	Bitter

Traditional Oriental diagnosis

A practitioner takes note of a patient's constitution, disposition, history, and lifestyle as well as any obvious symptoms in making a diagnosis. The four traditional methods used to obtain this information are looking, asking, listening and smelling, and touching (see facing page). Each method adds valuable insights from which a pattern emerges. Look for the particular patterns of disharmony in your partner to guide your own approach to treatment.

Facial diagnosis

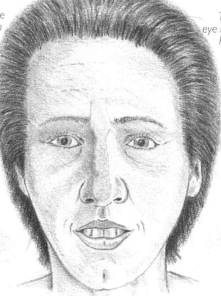

Head hair indicates a Kidney condition. Premature balding or greying shows deficient Kidneys.

The brightness of the eyes relates to the Mind and Essence – the constitutional strength of Heart and Kidneys. If the eyes shine the person has "good spirit" and can recover even from a serious disease.

Dark swellings under eyes result from weak Kidneys.

The colour of the upper cheek relates to the Heart and the Fire element. Puffy upper cheeks indicate a weak Small Intestine.

The colour of the lower cheek relates to the Lungs and the Metal element. Sagging lines or puffiness suggest a weak Large Intestine.

The colour of the tip of the nose is a Spleen indicator.

Lips and mouth are part of Stomach and Spleen function. Dry red lips and bleeding gums indicate Stomach Heat. Pale lips are the result of weak Spleen or weak Blood.

Sheen of hair reflects the health of the Lungs. Dull or brittle hair indicates weak Lungs.

A short chin indicates constitutionally weak Kidneys. A strong chin suggests a strong constitution.

Deep frown lines may indicate a temperamental, Liverish disposition/constitution.

The colour of the upper lid relates to Spleen; lower lid to Stomach.

The colour of the corners of the eye relate to the Heart: red means Heat; pale means weak Blood.

The iris and whole eye is part of the Liver function. Red eyes mean Liver Heat. Other eye troubles suggest a weak Liver.

The whites of the eyes reflect the Lungs. Red indicates dryness and Heat. Yellow indicates phlegm.

Bridge of nose area can reveal Liver and Gall Bladder disorders.

Ear lobe indicates the constitution and strength of Kidneys. Long and full ear lobes are a mark of strength and vice versa.

The teeth are part of the Kidney function. Weak, loose, or "dry" teeth suggests a Kidney deficiency.

Facial diagnosis

Facial diagnosis is widely practised in the Orient by doctors and fortune tellers alike. Many different systems and interpretations have developed since classical times and this can easily confuse the beginner. Only the most commonly accepted aspects are given here (see left).

The colours of the complexion give a general guide to the condition of the body. Red indicates overactive Yang or Heat, while pale or white areas show weak Ki and Blood, poor circulation, and Cold. A bright or shiny complexion shows a Yang condition. This is less serious than a Yin depletion indicated by dull, dry, or lifeless colouration. For the relationship between the colour of the areas of the face and the Five Elements, see the chart on page 25.

Looking

The general build, posture, and way of moving gives us insight into a person's constitutional vitality and attitude to life. A thin, wiry person will tend toward overactive Yang Ki, which can lead to exhaustion. Heavier, obese people may have weaker Ki and suffer from poor circulation and digestion. Any strain in posture reveals compensating or defensive Ki, always at the expense of another part of the body (see pp. 162–3).

More detailed observation of the skin, face (see left), eyes, tongue, and other parts of the body also form an important part of traditional diagnosis.

Asking

Straightforward, attentive inquiry after the details of a person's condition is an important diagnostic method. Begin with the onset and duration of any current problems and the person's general health and history. Then ask about the location of any pain or other symptoms that may indicate which Organs and Channels are involved. Ask about feelings of cold, heat, or feverishness and find out if the person is tired and lethargic, or nervous and restless. This indicates the balance of Yin and Yang as well as the overall energy levels. Other details, ranging from appetite, digestion, and excretions, to mood, occupation, and lifestyle help us to picture the disharmony.

Listening and smelling

Listening and smelling constitute one method in traditional diagnosis. The strength of the voice relates to the Lungs and indicates the strength of a person's Ki. The Heart and Mind influence coherence of speech. Wheezy breathing indicates phlegm (Damp), while quick, shallow breaths show depletion of Heart and Lung Ki. The sound of a cough tells us whether the Lungs are affected by Dryness or Damp.

The "Five Sounds" of the Five Element chart (see p. 25) relate to the expression of emotion as well as a quality of voice.

Subtle body odours are not easy to interpret. At the most simple level, a strong smell from perspiration or other excretions indicates a "Hot" disease.

Touching

The practice of shiatsu naturally places a strong emphasis on diagnosis through touch. Feeling for tsubos and learning to "listen" with your hands are dealt with throughout this book. You can obtain more information about your partner by feeling and pressing various parts of the body for comparison, examining the Channels and areas of pain for differences of temperature, resistance, and reaction (see pp. 162–3). Even more important is feeling the subtle qualities of the pulse and abdomen, or Hara. In Chinese medicine pulse diagnosis is the most important and profound diagnostic tool, but the Japanese have also developed Hara diagnosis to a refined level. Basic Hara diagnosis is introduced later in the chapter (pp. 164–5).

Touch diagnosis - kyo and jitsu

Stresses from the outside and within create distortions of Ki in the Channels. Distortions are always present to some degree as a result of day-to-day demands on the body. The quality of the body tissues changes, and tenderness or numbness, muscle tension or flaccidity, or stiffness or looseness in the joints may result.

Two Japanese terms, "kyo" and "jitsu" express the dynamics of this process. Kyo is the primary distortion, a "need" or emptiness. Jitsu is the compensating response that seeks to fill the need. For example, when you feel hungry (kyo) you make yourself a meal (jitsu) to satisfy your hunger. Practise feeling the difference between kyo and jitsu conditions in your partner, and treat according to the principles outlined on this page.

Kyo and jitsu in acute illness

When the needs of a kyo condition cannot be met, the body becomes vulnerable, and a defensive jitsu reaction covers the kyo condition. This complicates the job of finding the distortion. It may be helpful in acute cases to "sedate" or "disperse" jitsu areas and Channels. Apply a strong pressure for a short duration.

The body's reserves may be able to "fight off" acute illness, or compensate for an invading influence. Afterwards, however, the body will need time to recover and there will be a kyo aspect needing replenishment.

Kyo and jitsu in chronic illness

If distortions persist, chronic illness may develop, with both kyo and jitsu manifestations. The kyo aspect will display internal weakness, under-functioning Organs, and a corresponding flaccidity or emptiness in the Channels. The jitsu aspect shows itself as reactive tension, pain, or other superficial symptoms. You may be tempted to massage the jitsu aspects, but the traditional approach is to treat the primary, kyo, distortion with penetrating pressure. This tonifies the points and Channels by bringing Ki and Blood to deficient areas, thus filling the "need". It also releases Ki from the compensating or blocked areas.

Chinese laws of diagnosis

The applications of kyo and jitsu suggested here are a simplification of classical Chinese laws of diagnosis and treatment. These recognize, firstly, that illness occurs at different depths in the body; secondly, that you should find out and treat the "root" of disease rather than its manifesting symptoms. Thirdly, as a rule, you should tonify kyo conditions – inner deficiences of Ki and Blood – as a priority over dispersing excesses and blockages.

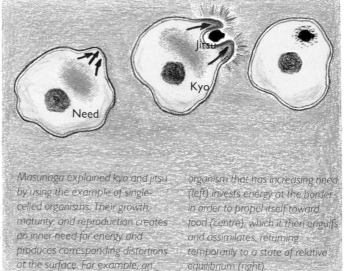

Masunaga explained kyo and jitsu by using the example of single-celled organisms. Their growth, maturity, and reproduction creates an inner need for energy and produces corresponding distortions at the surface. For example, an organism that has increasing need (left) invests energy at the border in order to propel itself toward food (centre), which it then engulfs and assimilates, returning temporarily to a state of relative equilibrium (right).

KYO AND JITSU IN THE CHANNELS

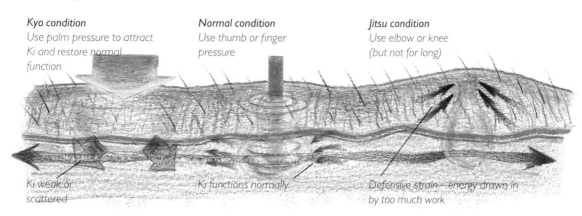

Kyo condition
Use palm pressure to attract
Ki and restore normal
function

Normal condition
Use thumb or finger
pressure

Jitsu condition
Use elbow or knee
(but not for long)

Ki weak or
scattered

Ki functions normally

Defensive strain – energy drawn in
by too much work

Tsubo wide open

Tsubo open

Tsubo closed
Hidden kyo condition.
Ki is difficult to reach,
and cannot be treated here

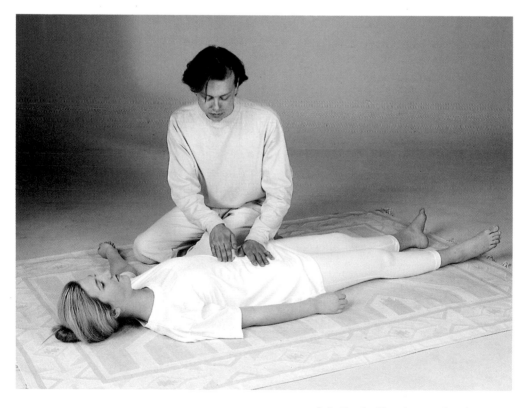

Palpating the Hara (see next page)

Focusing on the Hara

Hara diagnosis is used in Japan as an aspect of touch diagnosis. As with pulse, tongue, or facial diagnosis (see p. 160), it takes much practice to perfect.

Hara work reveals useful information about the condition of the receiver. As your touch becomes more sensitive and your understanding develops, you will learn to interpret what you feel. But always retain an open, or "beginners" mind; otherwise you will only pick up a reflection of your preconceptions.

Hara diagnosis depends on the breath reaching the Tanden. If tension blocks the breath, Ki from the Lungs will not reach the Hara and so it will not function as a vital centre. This makes detailed diagnosis difficult or even impossible.

Sitting by your partner's side to work with the Hara, you have the chance to combine all the other methods of diagnosis – looking, asking, and listening, with your touch.

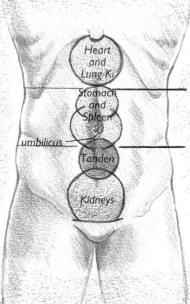

Simple Hara diagnosis distinguishes two main regions of the Hara: the upper and the lower. The upper region, between the ribs and the navel, should feel soft, flexible, but lively. The lower region, below the navel and including the pubic region, should feel firm and strong.

Another interpretation of the Hara regions divides them in the same way as the Triple Burner (see right). Masunaga developed a refinement (see far right) which differs in detail, but shares similar features.

Heart and Lung Ki

Stomach and Spleen

umbilicus

Tanden

Kidneys

Hara diagnosis, following the "Triple Burner" regions

The upper region should feel supple, free, and unconstrained.

Around the navel should feel lively, flexible, and responsive, not hard or soggy.

The Tanden "receives and stores" and should feel firm and strong.

Learning from the Hara

By gently feeling the Hara, you can obtain information about the Organs and Channels, using the guidance on the facing page. To interpret what you feel, you will need to develop your sense of kyo and jitsu qualities (see pp. 162–3). Try to develop an unobtrusive approach to working on this region. Your partner may feel protective about the area, but by your actions will be reassured.

Palpating the Hara

To palpate the Hara, keep your fingers extended but relaxed, and use perpendicular pressure from the weight of your relaxed arm. No further leaning is necessary. Don't push or press. Encourage your partner to relax, heed their breathing, and "listen" with your fingers.

Rest your near hand, palm down, on your partner's Hara, with the heel of your hand below the navel and your fingers above. Relax your shoulder and elbow. Initially, just slide your other hand gently under the arch of your partner's back. The tighter the muscles, the more arched the lumbar region will be.

Then, bring your hand from the back to support the upper Hara. With your near hand, gently probe the abdomen above and then below the navel with your fingers extended.

Note the general tonal quality and how the breath moves in the Hara.

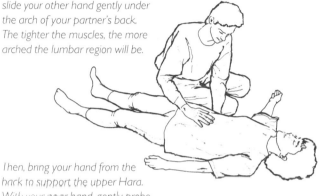

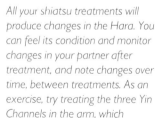

All your shiatsu treatments will produce changes in the Hara. You can feel its condition and monitor changes in your partner after treatment, and note changes over time, between treatments. As an exercise, try treating the three Yin Channels in the arm, which strongly influence the breath and emotional energy. You can treat them all with your partner in the supine position. The illustrations below remind you of the arm positions that expose each of the Channels most readily for your work.

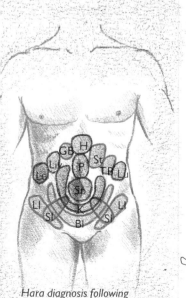

Hara diagnosis following Masunaga's arrangement

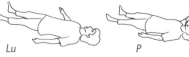

Lu   P   H

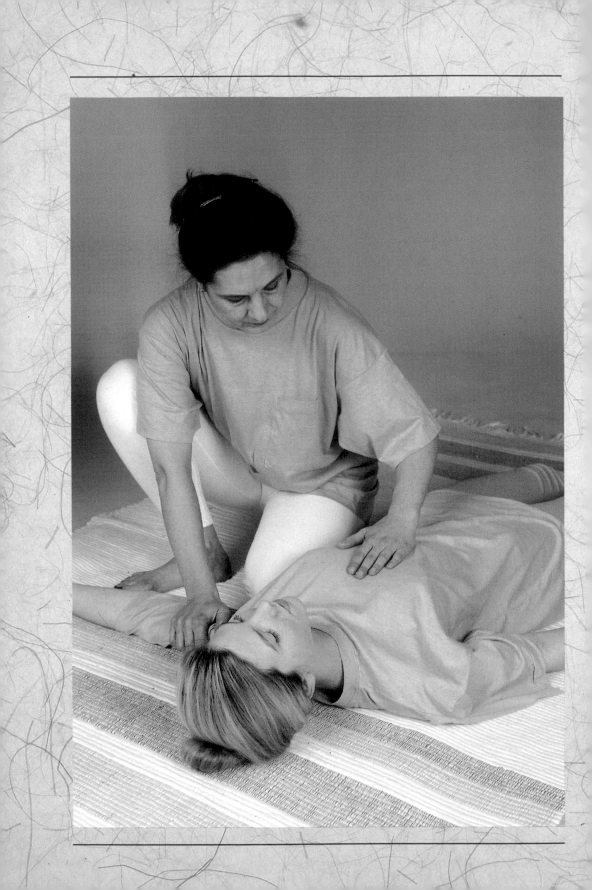

CHAPTER TEN

Everyday Shiatsu

As you become familiar with the shiatsu routines that are demonstrated in Chapters 4, 6, 7, and 8, you will gain the confidence to adapt the routines to suit the particular needs of your partner. Having learned the basic techniques and Channel pathways, you can adopt a more versatile approach in your shiatsu sessions. This chapter explores some of the ways in which you can use your knowledge of the Channels to develop routines for particular ailments or for the circumstances of everyday life.

The short routine for the head and feet given on pages 168–73 is suitable for treating people who are tired, over-stressed, and who cannot relax or sleep well. It is relaxing for the giver as well as the receiver, and can be done at the end of a busy day. Young children and pregnant women can also benefit from shiatsu treatment: follow the routines adapted to their special requirements on pages 174–7.

For those people who are uncomfortable lying on their front, or those who are not happy lying down at all, try the routine for shiatsu in the sitting position (see pp. 178–85). Use this for giving shiatsu to an elderly relative, or for treating a friend with asthma, or a colleague with a headache while you are at work. Each of these may prefer to sit either on the floor or in a chair.

Try to follow the principles of advanced technique, sometimes known as the "inner" principles (see pp. 52–54), and you will be able to adapt your shiatsu sessions to working on your partner in the sitting position and to any of the other demonstrations in this chapter.

Knowing how to adapt your shiatsu sessions not only helps you work with greater confidence but it develops an easy way with touch that positively enhances the richness and quality of your life.

Shiatsu for the head and feet

When people are tired, tense, agitated, and unable to relax, they are manifesting a Yin-Yang disharmony.

If Yin becomes too weak to attract and hold the Yang, or Yang becomes too strong in the body, the Yang separates and "rebels" upward. Headaches, nervousness, irritability, restlessness, insomnia, dryness of the eyes, nose, or throat, thirst, hot feelings in the chest or head, and flushed cheeks are typical symptoms of this kind of imbalance.

Giving shiatsu to the head and feet is often helpful in these circumstances. The routine lasts only 15 or 20 minutes. Try it at the end of a working day, or just before bed time, when its benefits will be most useful.

Begin with the head to disperse the Yang Ki and help it descend. Then work at the feet to strengthen the Yin, which attracts the Yang down. The Yin ascends to calm the Mind, cool the head, and moisten the eyes and throat. It helps the eyes to close at night.

The role of Yin and Yang
Yin attracts Yang; Yang attracts Yin. Yang is active and protects Yin; Yin nourishes and supports Yang. Yang is warm and drying; Yin is cool and moistening.

Yang Ki regulates the sensory "openings". The Yin Channels carry nourishment and moisture upward to the sensory orifices.

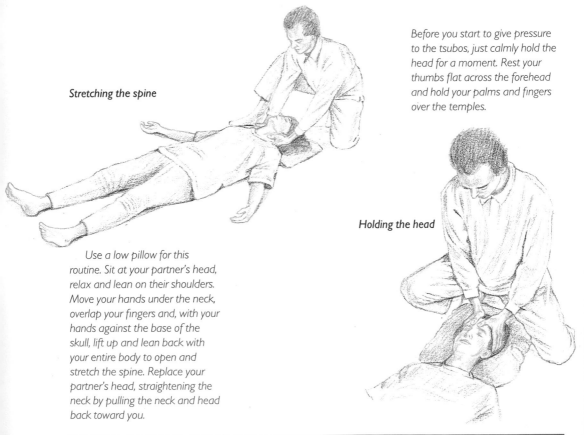

Stretching the spine

Before you start to give pressure to the tsubos, just calmly hold the head for a moment. Rest your thumbs flat across the forehead and hold your palms and fingers over the temples.

Holding the head

Use a low pillow for this routine. Sit at your partner's head, relax and lean on their shoulders. Move your hands under the neck, overlap your fingers and, with your hands against the base of the skull, lift up and lean back with your entire body to open and stretch the spine. Replace your partner's head, straightening the neck by pulling the neck and head back toward you.

Start by working on both sides of
the face at once. The symmetry of
your thumb pressure will feel quite
appropriate and comfortable as
long as you maintain support with
your extended fingers at the side
of your partner's head.

Use your thumbs to follow
the Bladder Channel up over the
forehead from the inner corner of
the eyebrow (Bl 2) toward the top
of the head. Next, follow the inner
line of the Gall Bladder Channel
from GB 14 up and over the head.
Then, using one thumb over the
other, follow the Governing
Channel from "Seal Hall", the
point between the eyebrows, up to
the top of the head.

It is not necessary to follow
the Channels rigorously. Try
working along the eyebrow line;
then follow the contours of the
face, below the eyes and across
and under the cheek bones.
Finally, work round the line of the
jawbone, using the thumbs on top
and curling the fingers under the
chin. Any tsubos that you find
relate to the Yang Channels on
the face (see pp. 76–7); but there
may be some classical points that
you feel will be particularly useful
for your partner. Feel free to
concentrate on them as you
come to them.

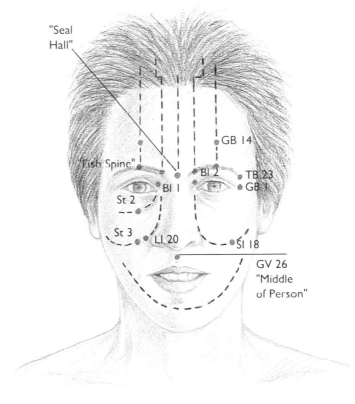

Working on the face

"Seal Hall"
"Fish Spine"
GB 14
Bl 2
TB 23
GB 1
Bl 1
St 2
St 3
LI 20
SI 18
GV 26
"Middle of Person"

The eyes

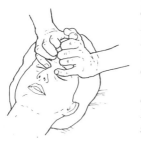

Work with the thumb is sometimes
difficult; use the little finger for
Bl 1, "Eye Brightness", which also
helps insomnia. This point is ⅒in
(1mm) above the inner corner of the
eye. Press inward and upward.

Points around the eye socket
are particularly useful for eye problems. Some also help in nose and
sinus trouble and most relieve head-

aches, too. These are annotated in
the above diagram and include "Fish
Spine", located in the middle of each
eyebrow; "Seal Hall", between the
brows on the mid line Channel; and
GB 14, "Yang White", 1in (2cm)
above "Fish Spine", which marks
the beginning of the inner line of the
Gall Bladder Channel over the head.

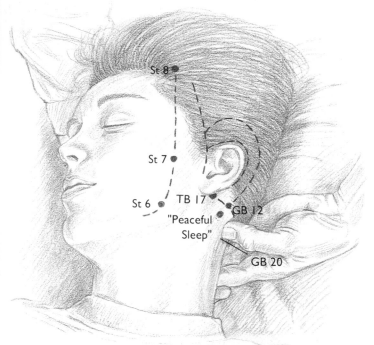

St 8

St 7

St 6 TB 17
"Peaceful GB 12
Sleep"

GB 20

Working on the side of the head and the base of the skull

After working over the face turn the head a little to the side, rolling it into your palm for support.

Now work down the side of the head, first thumbing the Stomach Channel from the corner of the forehead down in front of the ear to the muscle at the corner of the jaw. Then systematically work the tsubos along and within the hairline and around the ear. Finish by finding the tsubos under the base of the skull (see left). Feel for any hollows where your pressure feels accepted. Some of these are classical points with known benefits for the eyes, ears, and other sense organs. Some also calm the Mind and so are useful for insomnia, nervousness, or irritability.

Three-way stretch

This helps loosen and balance the neck. Roll your partner's head from side to side to feel for any resistance. If each side feels the same, begin on either side; otherwise, stretch the easy (kyo) side first (see p. 162).

Roll the head to face right, lean on the left shoulder with your right hand, and bring your left palm across to the side of the head (Position 1). Stretch the neck by leaning gradually into your hands, elbows relaxed, then release.

Reach your left hand behind the head to lift and turn it a little further (Position 2). Stretch and release. Then allow the head to roll back on to your palm, and stretch again (Position 3). Release. Repeat on the other side.

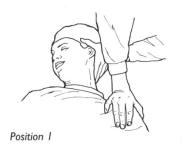

Position 1

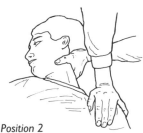

Position 2

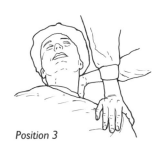

Position 3

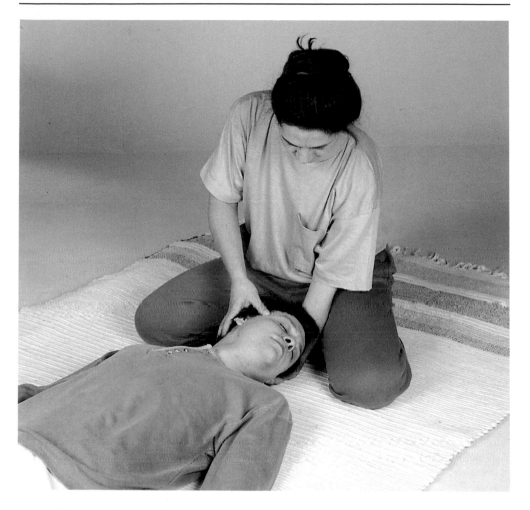

Working the Stomach Channel on the side of the face

Roll the head to the centre. Curl your fingers under the base of the skull and pull back slightly for a few moments, supporting the sides of the head with your palms. Then let your fingers find another position, penetrating the softer tissues or hollows (tsubos), and pull back again. Repeat this 2 or 3 times, allowing your partner to adjust, breathe, and relax each time. Then gently break contact and move to the feet.

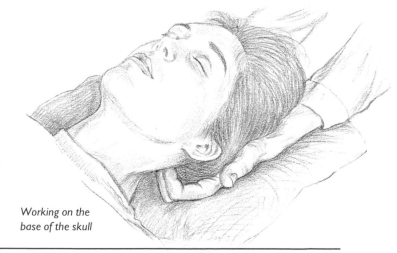

Working on the base of the skull

171

Treating the feet

Many of us spend much of the day on our feet. "Taking the weight off our feet" or "putting our feet up" are powerful metaphors for relaxation, and relaxation enhances their practical benefits. To work at someone's feet is also a true metaphor for the humble service we offer.

Work on the feet can affect the whole body, harmonizing Yin and Yang via the Channels as described already (see p. 168). The recently rediscovered system of reflexology confirms the ancient Chinese understanding that each part reflects and affects the whole.

Troubles of the feet and ankles, such as cramps, rheumatic pains, the effects of sprain, and other injuries can also be treated by careful shiatsu around the affected area and to nearby tsubos.

Rotating the ankle

Kneel by your partner's feet and take one foot on to your thigh. Hold the ankle just above the joint. Rotate the foot slowly and firmly with the other hand, a few times in each direction. Steady your arm against your other leg (see above), and work with body movement, not muscle power.

If your partner is relaxed, you should see a slight movement as a visible wave through the body as far as the shoulders and neck which confirms the improved Ki flow between the head and feet.

Liver Spleen

Kidney

Thumb the Yin Channels on the feet - the Kidney, Spleen, and Liver Channels. Work from the ankle and heel along the inner aspect of the foot. Cross under the arch to the sole for the Kidney Channel and follow the other two to the inner and outer edges of the big toe. Grip and rotate the toe. Give stationary pressure to any tsubos that seem open or responsive.

Thumbing the Yin Channels on the foot

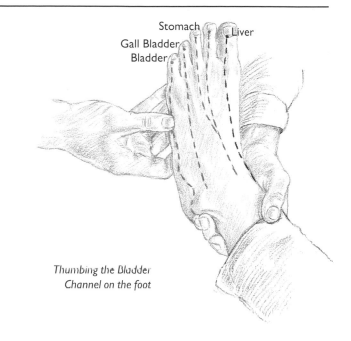

Stomach
Liver
Gall Bladder
Bladder

Change hands to work on the Yang Channels on the outer aspect of the foot. Begin with the Bladder Channel and work round the ankle and along the edge of the foot to the small toe. Then work the other Channels from the ankle points to the toes, feeling for the hollows between the bones and tendons. The Gall Bladder Channel goes to the 4th toe; the Stomach Channel has two branches, the main one going to the 2nd toe and another going to the 3rd toe, so work between all the bones.

Finish by stretching and rotating all the toes (see below).

Thumbing the Bladder Channel on the foot

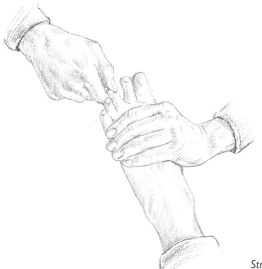

Finally, bend and stretch the whole foot in both directions, away from you by using your body weight to lean forward and bend the foot and toes back, then down, by grasping the top of the foot, as shown, and leaning back.

Change sides and repeat all the techniques on the other foot.

Stretching the foot

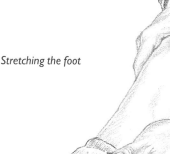

Note

The feet hold much tension and some people are quite sensitive about their feet. The effects of foot shiatsu can be powerfully releasing. Always be prepared to moderate your techniques and routines. Let your partner be your guide.

Shiatsu for children

Shiatsu with children can be formal or informal, a ritual at bedtime, or useful at any time. Children of all ages can benefit from shiatsu; and so, too, can parents. Shiatsu can literally help parents and children keep in touch with each other during the many phases of their developing relationship. It is not only an effective means of dealing with children's common minor ailments but a valuable way of reassuring them during illness, expressing feelings of commitment, and helping them to have trust in you. In many Oriental countries, children are encouraged to give massage to their parents when the day's work is finished. The children's valued contribution is a reminder of the reciprocal nature of family relationships.

On the whole, children are more Yang. They are prone to feverish or hot complaints, but their illnesses come and go quickly. They are sensitive and their Ki responds easily to pressure on the Channels and points.

Common ailments

In **fevers** *stroke repeatedly down the spine; down the Heart Channel to the small finger, and out from the bridge of the nose to the sides of the forehead. For* **poor digestion**, *often associated with* **teething troubles**, *give circular massage to the abdomen, and massage the thumb and forefinger, especially LI 4. Then massage St 36 and the Stomach line on the foot. For* **diarrhoea** *stroke up the Lung and Large Intestine Channels and massage repeatedly up the sacrum; for* **constipation** *massage down the sacrum. If the child is* **restless**, **irritable**, *or* **upset** *and* **panicky**, *try slow, steady massage of the palm, then grasp and gently squeeze along each finger to the fingernail. For* **bed-wetting** *and* **night fears** *rub the lumbar region to warm the Mei Mon. Hold the Hara and massage Kidney and Bladder points around the ankles.*

Massage for under fives

For very young children (0—5 yrs), rubbing or stroking along the Channels can be more appropriate and effective than pressure. Sometimes a combination of methods works well. Follow the general rule that you should massage away from the centre and down the limbs when the child is strong and fractious, or feverish and restless, with a loud cry or cough. When a child is weak, listless, or nervous, massage up the limbs and toward the centre. Refer to the back of this book for further reading on the natural treatment of children's ailments.

Stroke the chest — outward for an acute cough; inward from the ribs if the chest is weakened.

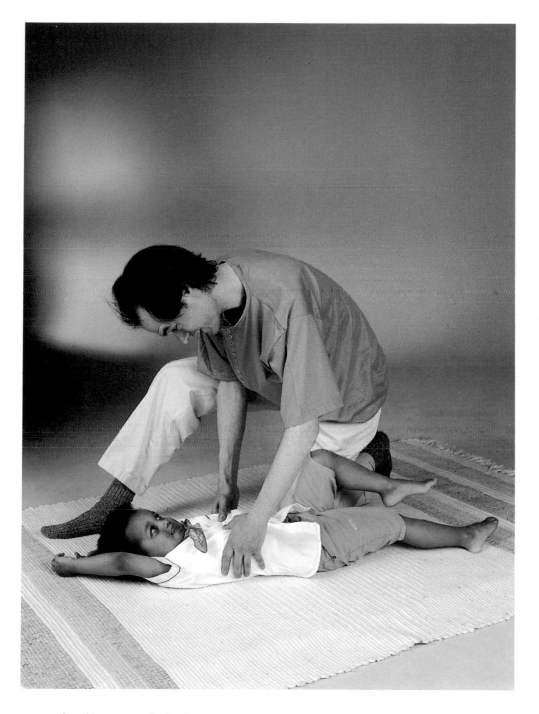

A stroking massage for the chest

Shiatsu for pregnancy

During pregnancy, a woman's body adapts to the new demands of nourishing and carrying the developing fetus. The mother's Kidney Ki and Essence are the principal sources of nourishment for the child growing within. The Kidneys are the root of Yin and Yang; typical symptoms in pregnancy are associated with the temporary loss of balance due to this diversion of Kidney energies. If the woman's constitution is weak, or if she is obliged to continue with strenuous work without sufficient rest, then the Kidneys (and hence other Organs), will be stressed, and symptoms may become persistent or serious.

Exercise, proper diet, and rest are all important. Shiatsu can be a great help, especially in the early and the later stages of pregnancy, as discussed below.

Exercises for pregnancy

Yoga classes for expectant mothers are sometimes available, but regular swimming is a good substitute, and the exercises given in this book can all be done quite safely, observing sensible limits.

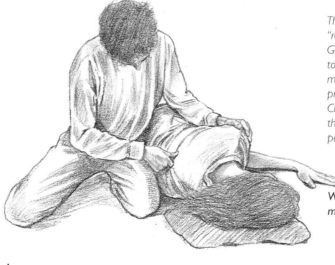

This condition, caused by "rebellious" Yang Ki of the Liver, Gall Bladder, and Stomach, is due to Kidney Yin depletion in the early months. Treat it by first giving pressure down the Bladder Channel with folded forefinger and thumb (as shown), with your partner in the side position.

Working the Bladder Channel for morning sickness

Cautions

Observe the cautions given on page 5 in this book concerning strong pressure on the Gall Bladder Channel at the top of the shoulders, and points LI 4 and Sp 6. Also avoid all the Yin Channels on the inside of the lower legs, if you are worried about the possibility of miscarriage in the early months. Other than this shiatsu is safe during pregnancy.

Treatment for morning sickness

The Bladder Channel affords a very balanced treatment in pregnancy: it helps the Kidneys and influences all the other Organs via their "associated points" (see p. 123). Concentrate on the middle region near the points for Liver, Gall Bladder, Spleen, and Stomach. Then give particular attention to the Pericardium Channel. Point P 6 is good for all sickness. On the Stomach Channel, work on St 36 and St 44. Lastly, give steady pressure to Liv 3.

One of the most common complaints in the late stages of pregnancy is lower backache and tired, heavy legs. The baby's weight puts strain on the mother's spine and a downward pressure on the pelvis. Haemorrhoids and varicose veins are the more severe manifestations of circulation impeded in this way.

As with the other conditions, all these symptoms can be helped by working on the Bladder Channel. Begin on the back and continue all the way down the legs, first palming, then thumbing. Lean in from behind as shown.

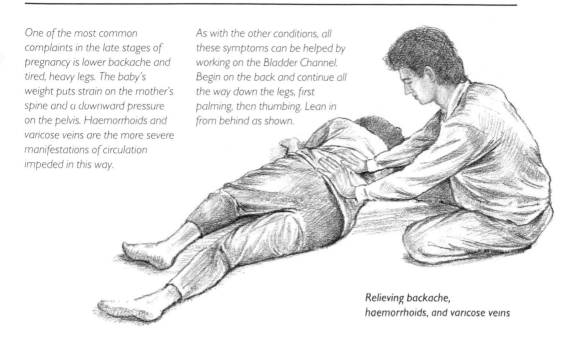

Relieving backache, haemorrhoids, and varicose veins

Shiatsu in labour can hasten and strengthen contractions and reduce pain. It can even bring on a delayed labour and save the need for artificial induction.

In giving shiatsu you should listen to your partner's needs, but generally your work should be strong - matching any pain when it occurs. All the forbidden points now become points of choice. Strong shiatsu on the shoulders often helps to start things off. Strong thumb pressure on the sacrum is often good when pains are bad. Try LI 4, Bl 60, and Sp 6, and give pressure to tender points on the ear.

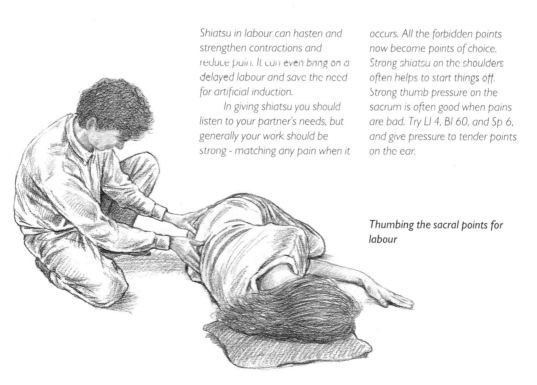

Thumbing the sacral points for labour

Shiatsu in the sitting position

You can practise shiatsu in any situation: it needs no preparation, only your versatility. Shiatsu in the sitting position is a useful means of treating people in everyday situations. But it is more than that. Elderly or disabled people may not be able to lie down easily; people suffering from asthma are often more comfortable sitting up, and it is a positive advantage to treat neck and shoulder pains or spasms in the upright position.

The major challenge of working on people in the sitting position is to provide them with support from your body while you work. Bring your leaning support into play. The routine that follows serves as basic practice, but soon you will be able to improvise and work in your own way.

Palming the back

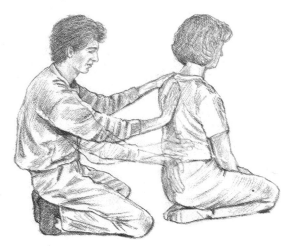

Beginning the routine
If your partner is able to sit comfortably on the floor, then this is the best place to work. Ask them to kneel or sit cross-legged and offer a cushion to make either position easier. Kneeling or sitting cross-legged for 15 or 20 minutes can be difficult if you are unused to it. Encourage your partner to move if they become cramped or numb. Adapt your work to a chair or stool if that seems best.

Begin by holding your partner's shoulder with your support hand and palm down the spine from between the shoulders to the sacro-lumbar region (see above). This allows you to feel your partner's condition, especially their breathing and any stiffness in the

spine. Relax your elbows and keep the pressure of your two hands equal and balanced.

Then move closer to support your partner's back as you give elbow pressure across your partner's shoulders from the corner of the neck (see right).

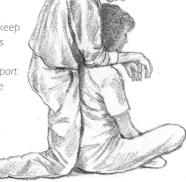

Leaning on the shoulders

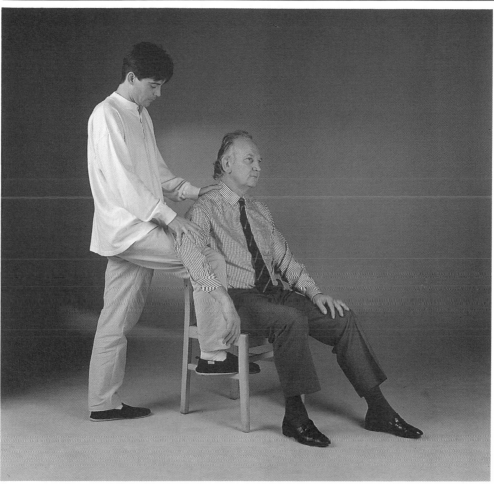

Working on the Triple Burner Channels on the shoulder

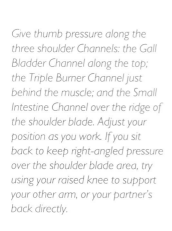

Give thumb pressure along the three shoulder Channels: the Gall Bladder Channel along the top; the Triple Burner Channel just behind the muscle; and the Small Intestine Channel over the ridge of the shoulder blade. Adjust your position as you work. If you sit back to keep right-angled pressure over the shoulder blade area, try using your raised knee to support your other arm, or your partner's back directly.

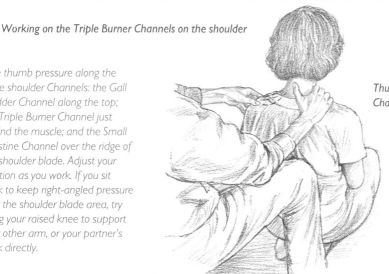

Thumbing the shoulder Channels

**Working on the Bladder and
Gall Bladder Channels to
clear the head**

In acute illness the Yang Channels
are called into play. Reacting to
external influences, Yang Ki produces
strong and unpleasant symptoms in
the head where the Channels meet.
Colds and sinus troubles, hayfever,
headaches, and hangovers, as well as
earache, and pain or inflammation
of the eyes are common.

Treat the Bladder and Gall
Bladder Channels, which run from
the eye region over the top of the
head. Their courses and connecting
links make them very effective in
dispersing blockage, clearing the
senses, and eliminating invasive climatic influences. Balance this local
work with shiatsu on the back and
limbs (see pp. 182–5).

Relaxing the neck

*Begin work on the head with this
effective loosening technique for
the neck. Move close and support
your partner with your thigh or hip.
Let your partner rest their head
forward on to your overlapping
palms. Keep your elbows on their
shoulders and give them time to
accept your support. Then raise
the head a little and slide the
hand touching the forehead out,
allowing the head to drop a very
short distance on to your other
hand. Catch them securely and
repeat a few times. Encourage
your partner to give up control.*

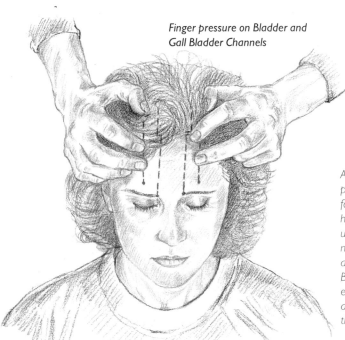

*Finger pressure on Bladder and
Gall Bladder Channels*

*After relaxing the neck, bring your
partner's head upright and lean
forward a little to support the
head gently with your body. Now
use your curled forefingers or
middle fingers to give pressure
along the Bladder, then the Gall
Bladder Channels, from the
eyebrows to the top of the head,
as shown. Don't "press". Rely on
the natural weight of your arms.*

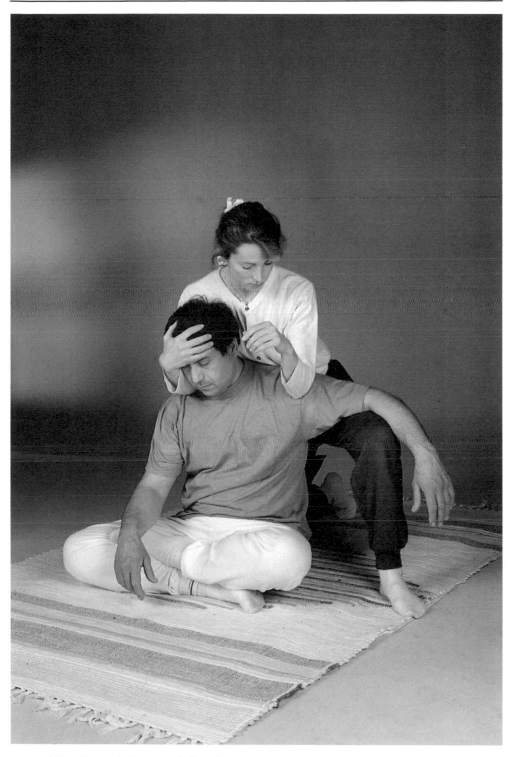

Using elbow technique to work down the arm

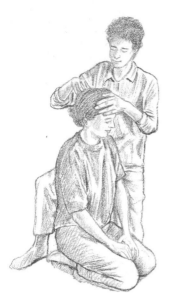

Bladder and Gall Bladder Channels from the side position

Move to the side, raise your knee to support your partner's back with your thigh, support the forehead with one hand, and continue to give pressure with the extended thumb and forefinger of the other. Work on the Bladder and Gall Bladder Channels over the back of the head.

Move your thumb and forefinger into the hollows at the base of the skull. Rotate the head gently with your support hand. Your thumb acts as a fulcrum at the base of the skull.

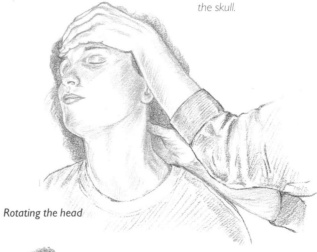

Rotating the head

Before you give shiatsu down the arm, rotate the arm at the shoulder to loosen the joints and help your partner relax. Move your supporting hand to grasp the shoulder of the arm that you are working with. For ease of control hold the arm just above or below the elbow and rotate it in widening circles a few times, forward, up, back, and down. Use your whole body, not just your arm muscles, to make the movements. Move out of your own way as you pull back. Go carefully through any stiff points. If you feel your partner helping or resisting, remind them to relax.

Shiatsu on the arm Channels
After a few full rotations bring your partner's arm to rest on your raised thigh, a restful position for you to use. Work down the arm using the palm, thumb, or elbow. The Large Intestine (see p. 181) and Triple Burner (see p. 179) are the most accessible Channels.

Rotating the shoulder

*Thumb and forefinger pressure
down the back*

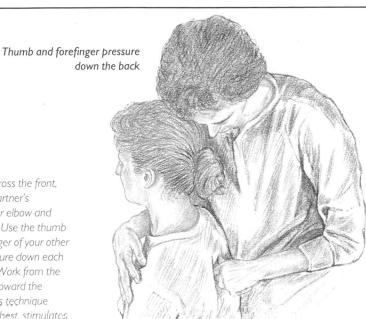

Place your arm across the front, supporting your partner's shoulders with your elbow and fingers (see right). Use the thumb and folded forefinger of your other hand to give pressure down each side of the spine. Work from the base of the neck toward the lumbar region. This technique gently opens the chest, stimulates the breath, and relaxes the whole back and spine.

Preparing for the full back stretch

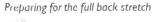

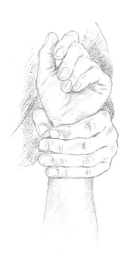

To prepare for the next technique, a dynamic back stretch, (see p. 185), stand behind your partner and clasp their hands firmly by the sides of the wrists, in the cleft between the bones (see left). A firm grip here prevents stretching the skin when you lift.

Make a number of preliminary rotations, carrying the arms up, back, and down again, reminding your partner to relax their shoulders and elbows.

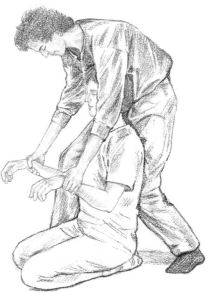

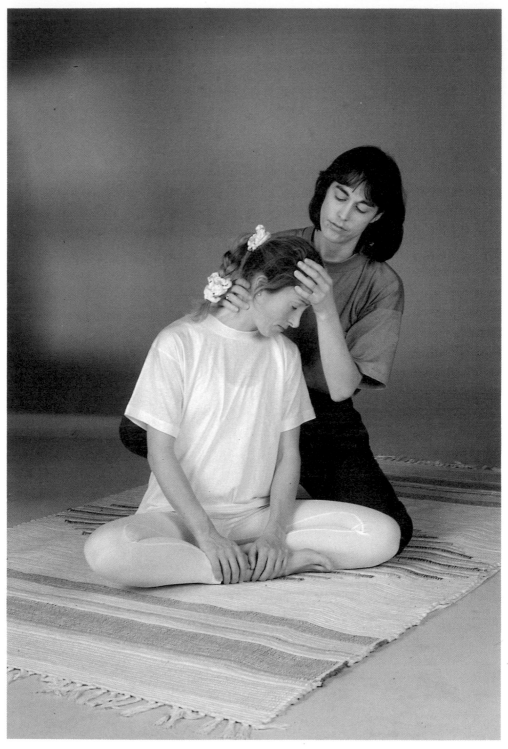

Rotating the head to loosen the neck

After one or two loosening
rotations, lift your partner's arms
up (see right). Find a suitable
angle to support the back against
your knee and thigh by adjusting
the position of your front foot, then
ask your partner to relax
backward, pause for a moment
and suggest they inhale then
exhale. On the outward breath
stretch your partner up and back,
using your knee as a fulcrum and
transferring your weight to your
back foot. Release the arms, circle
them round, adjust your knee up
or down a little, and repeat the
rotations once or twice.

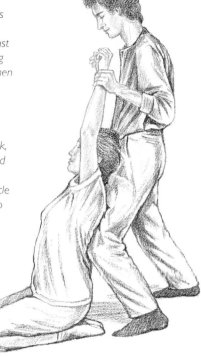

The full back stretch

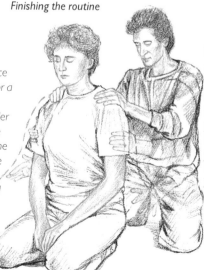

Finishing the routine

Replace your partner's arms on
their lap after the final stretch
and, kneeling down behind, place
your hands on their shoulders for a
moment. Let them settle. Then
squeeze and release the shoulder
muscles several times. Continue
this grip-release action across the
shoulders and then on down the
arms in quick succession. Then
"brush" down the shoulders and
arms to smooth the Ki.

Finishing the routine

After stretching and squeezing the
shoulders and arms, and brushing
down, it is, as always, best to finish
as you began. Sit back slightly, support one shoulder and give quiet contact in one or two places down your
partner's spine with your open palm.
Then they will feel settled. Let them
know that you have finished.

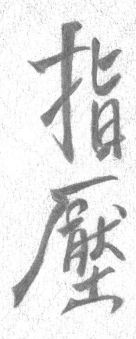

Shiatsu means relationship —
more than just "finger pressure".
Having hands we reach out to receive
and we extend ourselves in work.
Being heavy we need something to lean on,
the Earth lends us her body for support.
In shiatsu our partners lend their body for support.
Then, resting and strong, we can offer our hand in help.
Breathing Heaven's Spirit,
two people,
really one.

Index

Author's Acknowledgements

"Recognize, the grandfathers have said, that nothing unnatural exists. And that when man knows the truth, the whole truth, he gives name to that which he once called mystery; and that when a man needs to know something, a teacher appears."

Lakotah Indian
Hanta Yo: Clear the Way
Ruth Hill

Many teachers have helped me on my way and for their presence and guidance I offer my deepest gratitude. I would like to thank first of all, Bill Tara, who set my feet (and hands) on the shiatsu path, Gideon Ron, who nudged me forward, and Wataru Ohashi, for his inspiring early seminars in London. I am particularly indebted to Giovanni Maciocia who first laid out clearly for me the disciplines and wonders of Chinese medicine, and who has enhanced the knowledge and appreciation of this great subject in England.

I owe much to Michael Rose, Shinmei Kishi, and Pauline Sasaki, for their inspired and dedicated teaching. Special thanks are due to Pauline for her helpful criticism and cooperation.

I would also like to thank Helena Thomas, my first yoga teacher, whose Iyengar Institute in Brighton was a light in the darkness; Keith and Linda Codling for their guidance and healing sanctuary; Simon Wyard, my Tai Chi teacher, and Fabian Maman for teaching me Tao Yin Fa and Tama-Do.

This is an opportunity to record my heartfelt appreciation for the unique sense of commitment and support of the Shiatsu Society in Britain, and of my friends and colleagues there, whose warmth and comradeship I have been privileged to share. Thanks, especially to Elaine Liechti, its founding secretary, whose helpful comments on the manuscript of this book were gratefully received.

Thanks to all my students for their patience and commitment, particularly those who modelled for these pages; to my friend, Paula Cox, whose paintings eloquently enhance the interpretation of major themes; and to Eleanor Lines, my editor, and Dave Thorp, designer at Gaia Books, for their determination to see that, as far as possible, this book serves as an instrument for learning shiatsu.

Living daily with an author purporting to know something of the Tao, in fast-forward mode on his first book, can be something of an endurance. So my warmest thanks and love go to my family, to my two daughters Tamlin and Georgina who contributed their encouragement and practical support, and to my wife, Jacqueline, whose patience and understanding were sometimes stretched to the limit but who nonetheless did all she could to adapt to my inconsistent needs. Thanks finally, to our good friends, who quietly listened, supported, and offered their advice while this project was variously in or out of hand.

Publisher's Acknowledgements

Gaia Books would like to thank: Michelle Atkinson, Janine Christley, Eliza Dunlop, Lesley Gilbert, Jonathan Hilton, Libby Hoseason, Alison Jones, Danny McKenzie, Cass Pearson, Catriona Reid, Susan Walby, and Mary Warren for editorial and production work; Sara Firman for the index; Susan Berry, Chris Jarmey, (European Shiatsu School), Lucy Lidell, Elaine Liechti, and Pauline Sasaki for consultation; Marc Baum, Tim Crabtree, Bill Davis, Sarah Jarvis, Barbara Johnson, Jacki Jones, Evis Kleanthous, Gail Langley, Maurice Lavenant, Anamaria Lavin, Eleanor Lines, Sara Love, Georgina Lundberg, Tamlin Lundberg, Roger Newman, Veena Obrhrai, Ron Pallant, Nicholas Pole, Sam Pole, Michele Rogers, Ruth Sheldrick, Caroline Stevenson, Hedy Stute, Dave Thorp, Pam Thorpe, and Peter Warren for modelling. David Bruce Graphics Ltd, Tradespools Ltd, and Protocol Design Associates.

Bibliography

Beijing, Shanghai, & Nanjing Colleges of Traditional Medicine with The Acupuncture Inst. of the Academy of Traditional Chinese Medicine, *Essentials of Chinese Acupuncture* , Foreign Languages Press (China), 1980

Kaptchuk, Ted J., *Chinese Medicine: The Web that has no Weaver*, Century Hutchinson (UK), Congdon and Weed Inc. (US), 1983

Lao Tzu *Tao Teh Ching* (Lau D. C. English trans), Penguin (UK), 1963. (Feng, Gia-Fu & Jane English trans), Random House (US), 1972

Lo, Inn, Amacker, Foe, *The Essence of Tai Chi Ch'uan*, North Atlantic Press (US), 1979

Maciocia, Giovanni, *Foundations of Chinese Medicine*, Churchill Livingstone (UK and US), 1989

Masunaga, Shizuto with Wataru Ohashi, *Zen Shiatsu*, Japan Publications, 1977

Matsumoto, K. and S. Birch, *Five Elements and Ten Stems*, Paradigm Publications (US), 1983

Shangdong Medical College & Shangdong College of Traditional Chinese Medicine, *Anatomical Atlas of Chinese Acupuncture Points*, Shangdong Science and Technology Press (China), 1982

Shanghai College of Traditional Medicine (O'Connor, J. & D. Bensky, trans and ed) *Acupuncture: A Comprehensive Text*, Eastland Press (US), 1981

Veith, Ilza (trans), *The Yellow Emperor's Classic of Internal Medicine*, University of California Press (US), 1972

Wilhelm, R. (trans), *The I Ching or Book of Changes*, (Baynes, C.F. English rendition), Routledge Kegan Paul Ltd (UK), 1950

Wu, Zhang Ming & Sun Xingyuan, *Chinese Qi Gong Therapy*, Shangdong Science and Technology Press (China), 1985

Further reading

Chang, Jo Lan, *The Tao of Love and Sex*, Wildwood House, (UK), 1977

Chuen, Lam Kam, *The Way of Energy*, Gaia Books (UK), Simon & Schuster (US & Australia), 1991

Flaws, Bob and Honora Wolfe, *Prince Wen Hui's Cook: Chinese Dietary Therapy*, Paradigm Publications (US), 1983

Jarmey, Chris, and John Tindall, *Acupressure for Common Ailments*, Gaia Books (UK), Simon & Schuster (US), Angus & Robertson (Australia), 1991

Langre, Jacques de, *Do-In 2: The Ancient Art of Rejuvenation Through Self-Massage*, Happiness Press, (US), 1981

Scott, Julian, *Natural Medicine for Children*, Unwin Hyman (UK & Australia), Avon Books (US), 1990

Seem, Mark, *Bodymind Energetics: Towards a Dynamic Model of Health*, Thorsons (UK), 1987

Yamamoto, Shizuko, *Barefoot Shiatsu*, Japan Publications (Japan), 1979

Resources

For further study and training in shiatsu, contact the following:

UK

Shiatsu Society
c/o 14 Oakdene Road
Redhill
Surrey
RH1 6BT

USA

American Oriental Bodywork Therapy Association
50 Maple Place
Manhasset
New York
NY 11030

Australia

Australian Natural Therapists Association Ltd
PO Box 522
Sutherland
NSW 2232